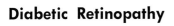

Diabetic Retinopathy

Diabetic Retinopathy

Edited by

John R. Lynn, M.D.

Chairman, Department of Ophthalmology
The University of Texas Southwestern Medical School
Dallas, Texas

William B. Snyder, M.D.

Department of Ophthalmology
The University of Texas Southwestern Medical School
Dallas, Texas

Albert Vaiser, M.D.

Department of Ophthalmology
The University of Texas Southwestern Medical School
Dallas, Texas

Grune & Stratton

A Subsidiary of Harcourt Brace Jovanovich, Publishers
New York and London

Library of Congress Cataloging in Publication Data
Lynn, John R.
  Diabetic retinopathy.

  Includes bibliographies.
  1. Diabetic retinopathy. I. Snyder, William B.
joint author. II. Vaiser, Albert, joint author.
III. Title. [DNLM: 1. Diabetic retinopathy. WK835
L989d 1974]
RE661.D5L9   617.7'3   74-1202
ISBN 0–8089–0820–0

Grune & Stratton, Inc.
111 Fifth Avenue
New York, New York 10003

Library of Congress Catalog Card Number 74-1202
International Standard Book Number 0-8089-0820-0
Printed in the United States of America

Figures 10-2, 10-6, 10-10, 10-12, 10-15, 10-28, 10-32, 10-35, and 21-3 are reprinted
with permission from Okun E, Johnston GP, Boniuk I: Management of Diabetic
Retinopathy; A Stereoscopic Presentation. St. Louis, Mosby, 1971, p 99, 69, 71, 77,
73, 87, 82, 85, and 46.

Dedicated to Kree, Phyllis, and Rebecca

With special appreciation to
Connie L. McAfee for her coordination
of both the meeting and the publication

Contents

Contributors

Francis I. Caird, D.M.
University Department of Geriatric
Medicine
Southern General Hospital
Glasgow, Scotland

Matthew D. Davis, M.D.
Division of Ophthalmology
University of Wisconsin Medical
Center
Madison, Wisconsin

Morton F. Goldberg, M.D.
Department of Ophthalmology
University of Illinois Teaching
Hospital
Chicago, Illinois

William L. Hutton, M.D.
Bascom Palmer Eye Institute
Miami, Florida

Eva Kohner, M.D.
Hammersmith Hospital
London, England

Francis A. L'Esperance, Jr., M.D.
Edward Harkness Eye Institute
New York, New York

Hunter Little, M.D.
Palo Alto Medical Clinic
Palo Alto, California

Lemuel T. Moorman, M.D.
Denver, Colorado

Edward Okun, M.D.
Department of Ophthalmology
Washington University School of
Medicine
St. Louis, Missouri

Arnall Patz, M.D.
Wilmer Ophthalmological Institute
The Johns Hopkins Hospital
Baltimore, Maryland

Gholam A. Peyman, M.D.
University of Illinois
Eye and Ear Infirmary
Chicago, Illinois

Marvin D. Siperstein, M.D.
Department of Internal Medicine
Southwestern Medical School
Dallas, Texas

H. Christian Zweng, M.D.
Palo Alto Medical Clinic
Palo Alto, California

Preface

When one reflects on the etiology of blindness throughout the world, trachoma is still the leading cause. An infectious disease, it can now be controlled by chemotherapeutic agents and antibiotics. Cataract is the major cause of blindness in the United States, but, like retinal detachment, it can be treated surgically. The remaining group of leading causes of blindness have membrane transport and/or blood flow deficiencies in common. This group includes glaucoma, senile macular degeneration, uveitis, and vascular retinopathies. Of these, diabetic retinopathy is the most frequent cause of permanent blindness. It is responsible for about five thousand new cases of blindness annually in the United States.

The papers collected in this volume were originally presented in 1972 at a symposium on diabetic retinopathy sponsored by the Department of Ophthalmology of the University of Texas Southwestern Medical School at Dallas. The authors represent all the major schools of thought on pathogenesis and therapy, and their contributions treat such topics as etiology and pathogenesis, current ophthalmologic therapy, and new approaches in research and diagnosis.

This book is not intended to offer final answers. Basic research is still needed to find an acceptable means of prevention and cure for diabetic retinopathy. However, we hope that this volume will add to the current store of information and, more importantly, stimulate further research into this major cause of blindness.

Marvin D. Siperstein

Chapter 1
Diagnosis of Diabetes

I have been asked to discuss the diagnosis of diabetes mellitus. I shall attempt to do so from the standpoint of the general internist who is faced with this very difficult and practical problem almost daily. There are few questions in endocrinology—or perhaps even in all of internal medicine—so confused today as that which asks, What is diabetes mellitus? Theoretically we define diabetes very simply. It is a genetic disorder characterized first by a relatively nonspecific abnormality in carbohydrate metabolism, ultimately by fasting hyperglycemia, and second, by a relatively specific form of vascular disease, the microangiopathy, which as it affects the eye is the major subject of this meeting. The microangiopathy of diabetes, in our view, represents, at least in the adult, the earliest and perhaps even the primary lesion of diabetes mellitus in that, by sufficiently sensitive techniques, one can consistently detect this lesion before the appearance of the earliest carbohydrate abnormalities of diabetes. But from a practical standpoint the endocrinologist is faced with diagnosing diabetes in the individual patient on the basis of the carbohydrate abnormalities of this disease. This in practice is remarkably difficult. I can illustrate the problem perhaps most dramatically by discussing the patient in Table 1-1, a 50-year-old airline pilot. During his yearly physical he unfortunately had a glucose tolerance test run. The fasting plasma sugar was found to be 125 mg/100 ml after 100 g of glucose; the 1 hour plasma sugar rose to 190; at 2 hours it remained at 130 mg/100 ml. A good internist had been told by almost every textbook and by the American Diabetes Association [1] that a glucose tolerance value at 1 hour of 160 or over, and a value at 120 at 2 hours or over, indicate diabetes mellitus in the face of a normal fasting blood glucose. The patient was told that he had moderate "chemical diabetes" since obviously these values exceeded the 160–120 mg/100 ml limits. The airline pilot was grounded since,

From the Department of Internal Medicine, The University of Texas Southwestern Medical School at Dallas, Dallas, Texas. Current address is the Department of Medicine, University of California Service, Veterans Administration Hospital, San Francisco, California 94121. This work was supported by USPHS AM 13866; Dr. Siperstein was the recipient of Research Career Award HE 1958.

Table 1-1

Results of yearly physical of 50-year-old pilot

FPS = 125	Dx: Moderate chemical diabetes
1 hr = 190	Rx: Grounded from flying;
2 hr = 130	Orinase 2 g/day

in the minds of the public and probably in the minds of his employers, a diabetic might develop diabetic coma at 30,000 feet. As noted he was also placed on tolbutamide 2 g/day.

This case illustrates two of the most common errors we see in diabetology. First, the diagnosis of "diabetes," "chemical diabetes," or any other type of diabetes in this patient is clearly wrong. Not even Dr. Fajans would consider this glucose tolerance test abnormal today. And, secondly, the treatment of such a normal person with Orinase or any hypoglycemic agent, especially with insulin, is obviously fraught with real danger. Even if the pilot did have chemical diabetes—and he doesn't—no one in the diabetes field, that I know of, would treat him with any oral hypoglycemic agent. This point is worth emphasizing because most physicians confuse chemical diabetes with overt diabetes. Chemical diabetes, even when a patient is so labeled, should only be treated with weight reduction if indicated, never with any pharmaceutical agent, insulin, or oral agent.

So, why was this normal pilot called "diabetic?" Why would many physicians treat his nonexistant disease? Why would many, in fact, make both errors? The basis of the problem lies in the widely publicized use of glucose values for an abnormal glucose tolerance test of 160 mg/100 ml at 1 hour and 120 mg/100 ml at 2 hours.[2] It is worth emphasizing that these data have never been published in definitive form and so we do not know the details of the "normal" subjects on which these figures are based. As a result of the broad acceptance of the "160–120" criteria for diagnosis of diabetes, many individuals in this country were labeled as diabetics. Table 1-2 presents some surveys of the incidence of diabetes that have appeared over the years.[3] If one takes patients over age 50, somewhere between 20 and 70 percent will be told that they have diabetes on the basis of glucose intolerance. This is obviously an error. Clearly, no one can really believe that half of our population over the age of 50 is diabetic. Nontheless, it is regularly concluded in such studies that this is the incidence of diabetes in patients with, for example, cancer or heart disease. Diabetics may be more prone to have large vessel disease, but the relationship is very hard to prove on the basis of the available data in the literature because of the recurrent use of the 160–120 criteria for diagnosing diabetes.

A simpler but still common problem that leads to the misinterpretation of glucose tolerance data results from the fact that most physicians do not realize that plasma or serum glucose values run 15 percent higher than those of blood; and a normal fasting serum or plasma sugar is not 110 mg/100 ml as we have been taught: it is about 127, which we round off to 130 mg/100 ml. So, if one finds a fasting plasma glucose value of 125 on a patient such as the pilot in Table 1-1, this is simply a normal plasma sugar.

Table 1–2

Incidence of Abnormal Glucose Tolerance Tests (Fajans-Conn Criteria) in Subjects Over Age 50

Normal, healthy, and dietary prep		Percent Abnormal GTT
Reaven		11
Brandt		15
Unger		35
Chessrow		22
	Average	21%
Patients, dietary prep		
Waitzkin		23
Streeten		46
Metz		39
Brandt		32
	Average	35%

Source: Seltzer HS: Diagnosis of diabetes. In Ellenberg M, Rifkin H (eds.): *Diabetes Mellitus: Theory and Practice.* New York, McGraw-Hill, 1970.

Secondly, the criteria of Fajans and Conn are certainly suspect in that they have never, to my knowledge, been confirmed. In 1957 Unger[1] attempted to define a normal glucose tolerance (Table 1-3). Note that upper limits of normal for plasma glucose tolerance in his extensive survey run about 100 mg/100 ml higher at 1 hour and at 2 hours than in the Fajans and Conn criteria. If one wishes to take a statistical definition of an abnormal glucose tolerance test, the figure therefore is not 160–120, but 260 and roughly 220 mg/100 ml. Note also that there is an age correction. As one progresses from age 20 to 50 there is a progressive increase in the glucose level after 100-g load of glucose at both 1 and 2 hours. Everyone who has studied glucose tolerance tests with 100-g glucose loads has confirmed Unger's original report.

Hayner *et al.,*[5] for example, examined 1-hour glucose tolerance levels in an

Table 1-3

Abnormal Glucose Tolerance Test
(Plasma)

Age	1 hour	2 hours
20–29	241	168
30–39	246	197
40–49	267	230
50–59	276	252

Source: Unger RH: Ann Intern Med 47:1138, 1957.

entire town. In the age group 40 to 59, well over half exceed the 160 mg/100 ml limit of glucose at 1 hour, and would be told that they are in the diabetic range. At a younger age the error is somewhat less, but is still an enormous 30 percent. The studies of Danowski et al.[6] have shown the same thing. All surveys that I am aware of have demonstrated that acceptance of values of 160 and 120 at 1 and 2 hours leads to absurdly high prevalence figures for diabetes mellitus.

The problem, then, is obviously that the initial concept of what is normal glucose tolerance is wrong. Fajans et al.[7] have implied this by recently introducing an age connection in what is a normal glucose tolerance test. Therefore, many individuals labeled "diabetic" a few years ago would now be called "normal." Whether an individual is diagnosed as being a diabetic depends not so much on whether or not he has the disease, but rather on the doctor he happens to chose.

The figures of about 260 and 220 should, as I noted, serve as the *statistical* definition of what is an abnormal glucose tolerance test. However, whether these figures have any *pathologic* meaning remains to be determined; for this reason we would be very reluctant to use even these statistical values for diagnostic purposes.

The other evidence that demonstrates prognostically that most glucose tolerance tests are worthless comes from the studies of O'Sullivan and Mahan,[8] who simply followed paients who had decreased glucose tolerance; extrapolating the result to 10 years, about three-quarters of these patients did *not* develop diabetes. In other words, the prognostic significance of an abnormal glucose tolerance test is extremely poor. We will therefore never tell the person that he is going to develop diabetes on the basis of any glucose tolerance test; certainly we will never tell the patient, as our airline pilot was told, that he *has* diabetes on the basis of this test.

In view of these studies it is safe to say that, unfortunately, the vast majority of patients who are today diagnosed as having diabetes on the basis of glucose tolerance data do not have diabetes and *never* will have diabetes. This is an extremely important medical and diagnostic point from several standpoints—both practical and theoretical. A decrease in glucose tolerance can result from many causes and is very nonspecific. Inactivity, that results from putting a patient to bed, will decrease glucose tolerance. Increasing age, as I mentioned, (perhaps due to relative inactivity), will decrease glucose tolerance. Obestity will decrease glucose tolerance. Perhaps the most overlooked of the current causes of reduced glucose tolerance is the use of contraceptive pills. Anxiety, through adrenalin release, will cause glycogen to be released, and insulin secretion to be depressed, and will result in a decrease in glucose tolerance. An airline pilot, with his high-paying job in danger, tends to be extremely anxious. He also tends to be inactive, obese, and aged, at least by the definition used here.

Fajans has always maintained that the glucose tolerance test should not be used in anyone who is sick. He has stressed that this test applies only to otherwise healthy, ambulatory subjects under the age of 50; it does not apply to individuals over 50 with any acute or chronic disease. Therefore, even by his criteria one cannot use a glucose tolerance test for any hospitalized patient. Though most patients who have glucose tolerance tests come to their doctor with some sort of acute or chronic disease, this admonition is often forgotten or ignored. Incidentally, there never were any good data to support the concept that a 300-g carbohydrate diet is necessary before a glucose tolerance test. Eating a normal carbohydrate diet results in the same glucose tolerance test as will 300 g of glucose a day; and diet can therefore rarely be invoked as the cause of a decrease in glucose tolerance.

So, no one in the field today should call the airline pilot in Table 1-1 a diabetic. But most physicians in practice would, and this is the practical consequence of the confusion surrounding the glucose tolerance test.

From the *theoretical* standpoint—from the standpoint of the individual studying diabetic retinopathy, carrying out epidemiologic studies, and seeing whether good control of diabetes prevents vascular disease—these data mean that unless diabetes is carefully defined, serious errors will result.

Most "chemical" diabetics will not develop retinopathy because they do not in fact have diabetes mellitus. If one then carries out a study to see whether good control prevents retinopathy, clearly there is no trouble in achieving excellent control in those patients who have chemical diabetes because the majority of them are perfectly normal. Since of course these subjects will never develop retinopathy, one will fall into a very common trap of saying that good control has prevented retinopathy. It is this *post hoc ergo propter hoc* reasoning that has tainted many studies of the effect of good control on the complications of diabetes.

The widely publicized University Group Diabetes Project,[9] which indicated that Orinase causes deaths from myocardial infarction, was seriously flawed by this mistake. A significant percentage of the "diabetic" patients in that study were not diabetic at all, even by the criteria that were set up for the study. Moreover, those criteria are not adequate to fulfill the statistical criteria of Unger. It is probably a safe extrapolation to say that at least 30 percent of the patients who were called diabetic in the University Group Diabetes Project did not have diabetes. Aside from the question of treating nondiabetic patients with tolbutamide or insulin, obviously a study of diabetic vascular disease tainted with 30 percent patients who are not diabetic at all produces a very questionable result.

So, if we conclude that the glucose tolerance test to date cannot be used as a valid means of diagnosing diabetes, how does one practically face the problem of telling a patient he does or does not have diabetes mellitus? Practically, we will not tell an individual that he has a glucose abnormality in the diabetic range until he has *consistent fasting* hyperglycemia—that is, a plasma glucose over 140 mg/100 ml at least twice. The usual cause of "fasting" hyperglycemia is that the patient has forgotten to miss breakfast. Consistent fasting hyperglycemia in the absence of the many diseases that will cause hyperglycemia besides genetic diabetes mellitus—i.e., pancreatitis, Cushing's disease, acromegaly, pheochromocytoma, and severe hyperlipemia—indicates diabetes. In the absence of these secondary causes of hyperglycemia, we will tell the patient he probably has diabetes mellitus. These, at least, are solid criteria.

Obviously, if one uses these criteria, he will miss some early diabetics. What is the harm in this? It is probably nil. No one, as I have indicated earlier, would treat such patients who have decreased glucose tolerance with any measure except diet. If they are overweight, we tell them to lose weight. We tell such a patient to come back in 6 months, and that he has a decrease in glucose tolerance; but we would never use the word diabetes.

What, then, is the damage done by overdiagnosing diabetes? It is enormous. The pilot loses his job. There are genetic implications in that his children will very probably be told that they carry a diabetic gene. If he has insurance, his rates will markedly increase. He is told he has a devastating disease which will lead, in 75 to 80 percent of the cases, to retinopathy in 15 to 20 years. And all of these consequences are unnecessary since there is no evidence that such a patient does in fact have diabetes.

This, then, is why the diagnosis of diabetes represents one of the major problems for the endocrinologist today. The message I wish to leave with you is that the diagnosis of diabetes mellitus by any measure of carbohydrate intolerance short of consistent fasting hyperglycemia, is fraught with error. Diabetes is not an easy diagnosis to make; it should be made with extreme conservatism. The harm of overdiagnosis is enormous; the harm of underdiagnosis is trivial. It is our view that until a better procedure is available, one should make the diagnosis of diabetes mellitus in an individual patient only when that patient has consistent fasting hyperglycemia.

REFERENCES

1. Standardization of the Oral Glucose Tolerance Test. Report of the Committee on Statistics of the American Diabetes Association, June 14, 1968. Diabetes 18:299, 1969

2. Fajans SS: Diagnostic tests for diabetes mellitus. In Williams RH (ed): Diabetes. New York, Hoeber, 1960, p. 397

3. Seltzer HS: Diagnosis of diabetes. In Ellenberg M, Rifkin H (eds): Diabetes Mellitus: Theory and Practice. New York, McGraw-Hill, 1970, p 436

4. Unger RH: The standard two-hour oral glucose tolerance test in the diagnosis of diabetes mellitus in subjects without fasting hyperglycemia. Ann Intern Med 47:1138, 1957

5. Hayner NS, Kjelsberg MO, Epstein FH, Francis T Jr: Carbohydrate tolerance and diabetes in a total community, Te-

cumseh, Michigan. Diabetes 14:413, 1965

6. Danowski TS, Aarons JH, Hydovitz JD, Wingert JP: Utility of equivocal glucose tolerances. Diabetes 19:524, 1970

7. Fajans SS, Levine R, Moss JM: The diagnosis of diabetes. Installment 4: Identifying the diabetes suspect. Gen Prac 39:141, 1969

8. O'Sullivan JB, Mahan CM: Prospective study of 352 young patients with chemical diabetes. N Engl J Med 278:1038, 1968

9. Klimt, CR, Knatterud GL, Meinert CL, Prout TE (prepared for the University Group Diabetes Program): A study of the effects of hypoglycemic agents on vascular complications in patients with adult-onset diabetes. I. Design, methods and baseline results. Diabetes 19(suppl): 747, 1970

Matthew D. Davis

Chapter 2

Definition, Classification, and Course of Diabetic Retinopathy

Laying some sort of a foundation is not as easy a job as one might think, for although we all know what diabetic retinopathy looks like ophthalmoscopically, it is difficult or impossible to define it in such a way as to exclude the similar fundus appearance sometimes seen in hypertension, severe arteriosclerosis, branch vein occlusion, dysproteinemias, and occasional rare retinal vascular anomalies. To classify diabetic retinopathy is also a difficult task. I will illustrate the various typical ophthalmoscopic lesions of diabetic retinopathy and the highly variable course which may be followed by them. The work which I will present is not mine alone, but is the product of a team consisting of Dr. R. L. Engerman, Dr. F. L. Myers, Dr. G. deVenecia, and Dr. G. H. Bresnick.

Diabetic retinopathy is conventionally divided by ophthalmologists into two major stages: nonproliferative and proliferative. I have serious reservations about the term nonproliferative, since I suspect that some of the lesions conventionally belonging to this stage do indeed represent proliferation of vascular endothelium. But I know of no better term. Internists, pathologists, and others with fundamental interest in the microangiopathy of diabetes object, and rightly so, I believe, to the term so many of us use, background retinopathy, as a synonym for nonproliferative. I am afraid I must accept a significant share of the blame for the coinage of this term, which is really only appropriate to the ophthalmologist who is studying or attempting to treat neovascular proliferations.

Although the relationship between them is not entirely clear, there are, I believe, at least four processes going on in diabetic retinopathy. These four processes are obliteration of retinal vessels, proliferation of endothelial cells and fibrous tissue, increased permeability of vascular walls, and contraction of the fibrous tissue and the vitreous to which it is related. Figures 2-1 and 2-2 illustrate the sort of retinopathy that the internist sees frequently and that the ophthalmologist does not see too frequently. I start out with this because, ophthalmoscopically, I think this is the beginning. I have never been convinced that venous dilatation prior to the appearance of microaneurysms is really a characteristic feature; but again, as an ophthalmologist, I do not routinely see a lot of very early patients.

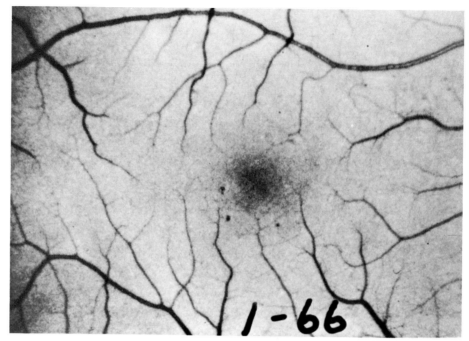

Fig. 2-1. Early diabetic retinopathy (cf. Fig. 2-2).

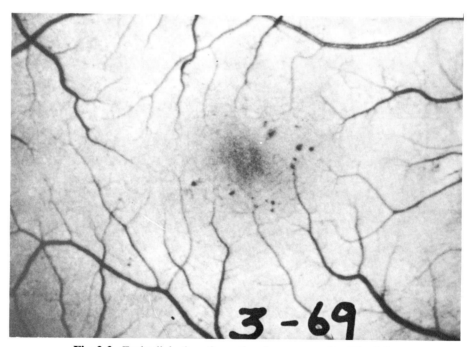

Fig. 2-2. Early diabetic retinopathy, three years after Fig. 2-1.

At any rate, this patient is fortunate in that he does not progress very much. He has a few red dots, probably all microaneurysms; more than 3 years later there is not very much difference. And of course, this patient is in no trouble. His vision is normal.

What other lesions are there in early diabetic retinopathy? In Figure 2-3 we see our familiar little round red dots—aneurysms—perhaps some of them are punctate hemorrhages. But there is something else present that is not very easy to see. I had to look through a lot of photographs to find something that would show. What I hope are apparent are two faint, soft exudates or cotton wool patches. There are also several slightly dilated little vessels. I think this is a fairly characteristic regional lesion of diabetic retinopathy, and I would suggest that there are obliterated capillaries in the center. I cite the soft exudate as evidence of vascular obliteration. This is what cotton wool exudates are—ischemic infarcts in the retina. I would suggest that the dilated small vessels which characteristically appear around the ischemic area represent attempts at neovascularization, attempts at endothelial proliferation in response to ischemia.

Figure 2-4 shows the histologic counterpart in a trypsin digest preparation from a different patient. The capillaries near the bottom of the picture have endothelial and pericyte nuclei. In the center the capillaries do not have any cells; I think most pathologists agree that this means they are indeed occluded and that no blood is flowing through them. Surrounding this area are microaneurysms, most of which, in this specimen, are highly cellular. Some have very thickened walls which stain intensely with PAS. Near the top of the illustration is one of these dilated, large caliber, very hypercellular channels that Dr. Cogan and Dr. Kuwabara

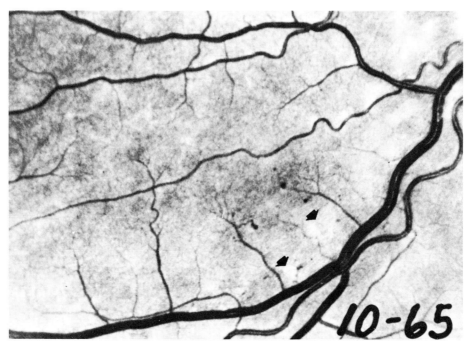

Fig. 2-3. Early retinopathy showing microaneurysm and two cotton wool spots (arrows) (cf. Figs. 2-5 and 2-6).

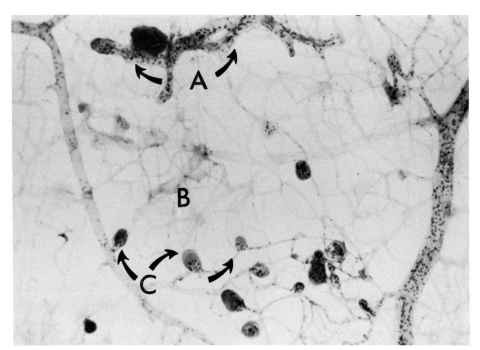

Fig. 2-4. Histology of early diabetic retinopathy. This trypsin digest preparation demonstrates shunt vessels (A), acellular capillaries (B), and microaneurysms (C).

have called shunt vessels. They have suggested that shunt vessels come first and that they usurp the blood flow from other vessels which then become obliterated. Although the matter, I think, is not entirely settled, I am inclined to agree with the majority of other people interested in this area that the obliteration probably comes first. And, if we agree with that, then we have two possibilities: either the blood flow is diverted and causes hypertrophy of these channels, or we might explain these dilated hypercellular channels the same way that I would like to explain microaneurysms, which is that they represent proliferation of the vascular endothelium in response to ischemia. If these were dilating to carry the extra load of blood that had to flow through them because other capillaries were obliterated, I think we would expect rapid flow. But, in fact, in fluorescein, as I think perhaps Dr. Kohner will show us later, and as is true in our experience, the flow is quite slow in these vessels. That is one of the things that leads me to feel that they are a response to ischemia.

Now I will show you what happened to the eye in Figure 2-3. Characteristically, the lesions in diabetic retinopathy change. We ophthalmologists are more likely to see patients when they change for the worse rather than when they change for the better. Actually, not infrequently changes occur in both directions at once. One part of the eye is getting better and one part worse.

In Figure 2-5 the soft exudates, aneurysms, and dilated vessels noted in Figure 2-3 can no longer be seen, but superiorly, near the disc, there is now a new soft exudate. Soft exudates are very common in relatively early diabetic retinopathy and, at this stage, at any rate, seem to be unrelated to hypertension. There was an excellent study done some years ago by Esmann et al.[1] documenting this very well. They found that the soft exudates were as characteristic of diabetic retinopathy as hard waxy exudates.

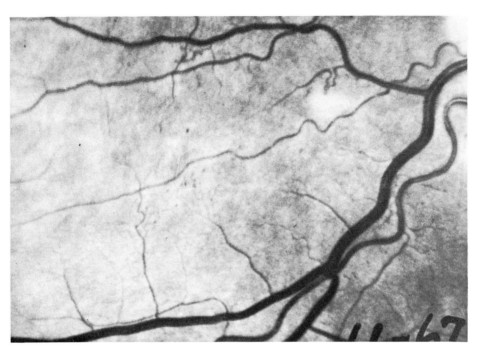

Fig. 2-5. Two years later the soft exudates, aneurysms, and dilated vessles noted in Fig. 2-3 cannot be seen, but superiorly, near the disc, there is now a new soft exudate (cf. Figs. 2-3 and 2-6).

Figure 2-6 shows the same area 1 year after Figure 2-5 and 3 years after Figure 2-3. The soft exudate present in Figure 2-5 has gone away, but the abnormal vascular channel, which was already beginning, is larger. I would suggest that the same thing is going on in this area that went on previously in the other area. Perhaps there has been so much obliteration of the circulation in the first area that the ophthalmoscopic appearance is better. My guess is that if we had a trypsin digest preparation we would see a lot of obliterated capillaries there.

Figure 2-7 shows an interesting patient whom we have followed for a number of years; I want to trace the evolution of this one aneurysm. In 1964 there was a rather large aneurysm with a fairly thick wall and a ring of hard exudate around it. If we were looking at this patient with a slit lamp, we would see a thickening of the retina resulting from retinal edema which characteristically occurs around a single aneurysm or a clump of aneurysms. Characteristically, one sees the hard lipid deposits around that. In Figure 2-8, not quite a year later, the aneurysm looks perhaps a little larger, but the exudates have gone away and probably the retinal edema has gone away too, although we really cannot tell that from the photograph. In Figure 2-9, 3 years later, the aneurysm is becoming rather difficult to see. The wall is becoming so thick that it is difficult for us to see the blood in the lumen. Yet in 1 year more (Fig. 2-10) apparently the wall has become so thick that we now just see a white spot; and whether or not there is still a lumen in the aneurysm, we cannot tell for certain. Figure 2-11 is a high-powered trypsin digest preparation to suggest the histologic counterpart. On the left is a thin-walled aneurysm without much PAS-positive material in the wall, and on the right a

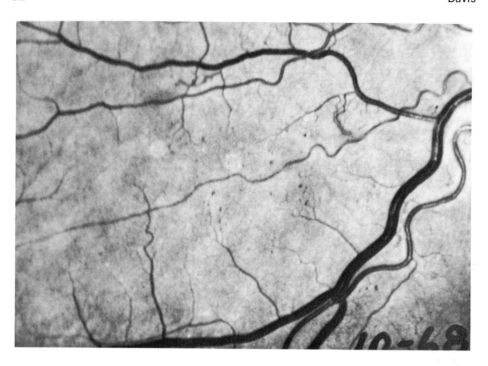

Fig. 2-6. Soft exudate of Fig. 2-5 has disappeared while abnormal vascular channel enlarges with intervening years (cf. Fig. 2-5).

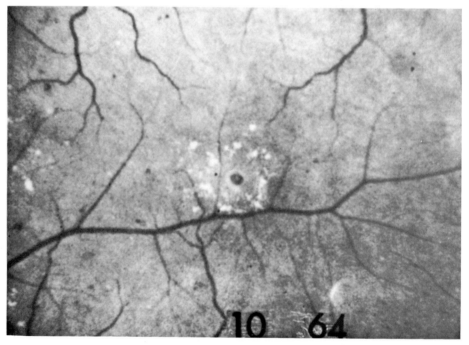

Fig. 2-7. Large retinal aneurysm with thick wall and ring of hard exudate (cf. Figs. 2-8, 2-9 and 2-10).

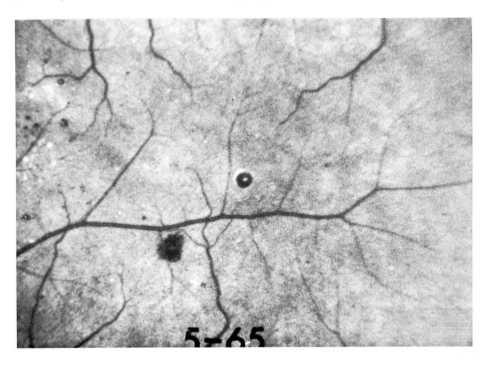

Fig. 2-8. Eleven months later the aneurysm of Fig. 2-7 has enlarged and the exudates have disappeared (cf. Figs. 2-7, 2-9 and 2-10).

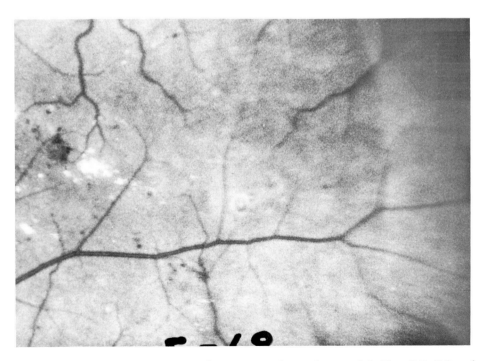

Fig. 2-9. After three more years, the aneurysm is poorly seen (cf. Figs. 2-7, 2-8 and 2-10).

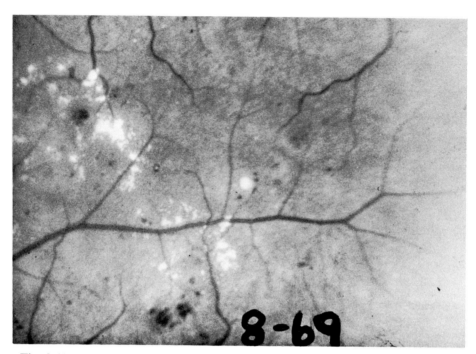

Fig. 2-10. One year later, the aneurysm appears as a white spot (cf. Figs. 2-7, 2-8 and 2-9).

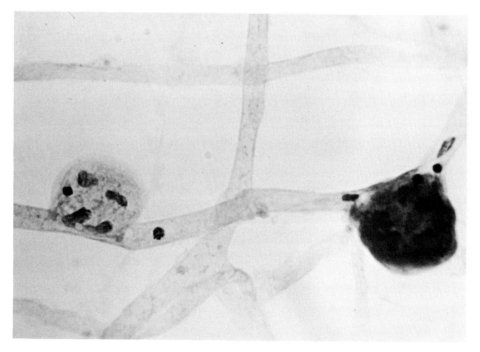

Fig. 2-11. The presumed histology of the aneurysm in Figs. 2-7 through 2-10. Earlier appearance on left; later stage on right (trypsin digest preparation).

thick-walled aneurysm. The aneurysm illustrated in Figures 2-7 to 2-10 progressed from the stage on the left to the stage on the right, and perhaps well beyond that.

Figure 2-12 is included to emphasize again one of the processes that was mentioned at the beginning, the leakiness of vascular walls. There are several thick- and thin-walled aneurysms in the center of the rings of the exudate. Actually there are three rings: a little one inferiorly and two larger ones above that. This is a very characteristic appearance, and we would easily see the thickening of the retina due to edema if we looked at this patient with the slit lamp. The retinal edema has been missed in the past, but I think enough people are talking about it now that you all know about it. But, 5 years ago or so it was very common, I think, in practice for this edema to be missed, because, as you can see, the retina is still transparent. You can see the choroid through it, almost normally. It is only with a stereoscopic method that one can see this marked thickening in the retina.

Figure 2-13 is another example of macular edema. These are three aneurysms with thick walls or a lipid deposit around them. We generally refer to this clinically as thick walls. I think that is what it is. But sometimes when there is a marked deposit like this, I wonder whether some of this material is not really outside the wall. This is a left eye; the disc is off the picture to the left, and there is a large cystic area in the macula. This leakiness is surely the most common mechanism involved in the moderate degree of visual impairment that diabetics with nonproliferative retinopathy frequently have.

Figure 2-14 demonstrates that macular edema is not always associated with rings of exudate. The typical polycystic spaces are difficult to see without stereo.

The appearance of some lesions makes me feel that a lot of what we are

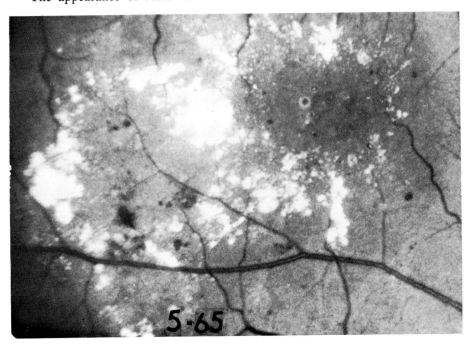

Fig. 2-12. Three rings of retinal edema and exudate surrounding leaky retinal aneurysms.

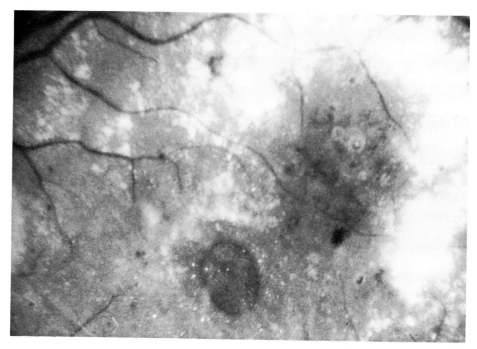

Fig. 2-13. Macular edema with three aneurysms and surrounding lipid deposits.

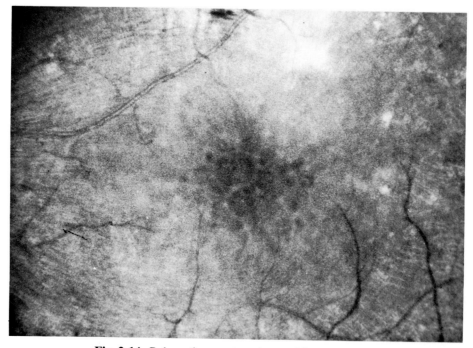

Fig. 2-14. Polycystic macular edema without exudates.

watching is vasoproliferation. Figures 2-15 to 2-19 are of the superotemporal quadrant of the left eye of a patient with juvenile onset diabetes. The macula is off the picture below; the disc is to the left. In Figure 2-15 we see many of the lesions of diabetic retinopathy. There are a few hard exudates, lots of blot hemorrhages, and some dot hemorrhages, or aneurysms. There are abnormal vascular channels within the retina. There has been a lot of controversy as to whether these represent new vessels—actual proliferation of new vessels within the retina—or whether they are dilatations of preexisting channels. This is a difficult question to answer; I think both viewpoints are true. When the vasoproliferative stimulus is strong enough, actual new vessels probably develop within the retina and then break through its internal surface. But at any rate, we do see these dilated channels for which the term intraretinal microvascular abnormalities has been used. I am not terribly happy with that term. It represents a begging of the question as to whether these are new vessels or dilated preexisting channels and, as you might imagine, our photographers and physicians' assistants soon abbreviate intraretinal microvascular abnormalities to IRMAs. Notice the beading of the retinal veins. Note the formation of a little loop, which looks as though the vein is trying to form another channel, just before the last upper branch of the superior temporal vein leaves the picture.

Three months later (Fig. 2-16) this vein appears "double-barrelled." We have called this "reduplication," for want of a better term. In Figure 2-16 faint, soft exudates are also present, one being fairly prominent. These appearances typically occur just prior to development of surface neovascularization. This whole process seems to go along slowly for awhile and then to reach a crescendo, as it were, and this is the point where we expect the cymbals to crash and new vessels

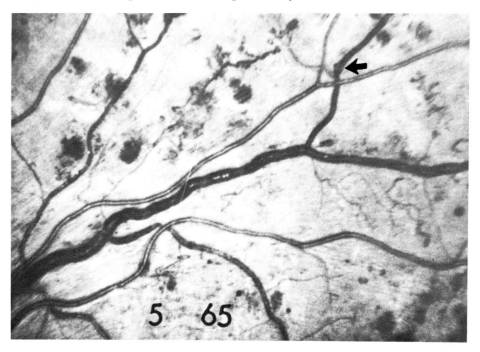

Fig. 2-15. More advanced retinopathy showing venous beading, intraretinal microvascular abnormalities (IRMA's) and a venous loop (arrow) (cf. Figs. 2-16, 2-17, 2-18 and 2-19).

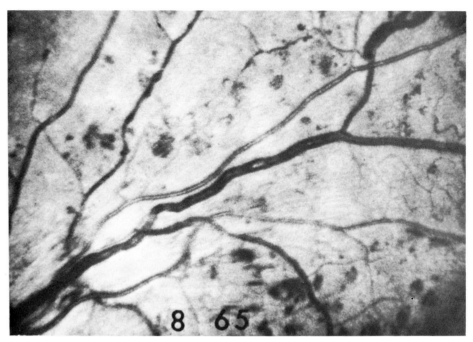

Fig. 2-16. Three months later venous reduplication has appeared in area of venous loop in Fig. 2-15 (cf. Figs. 2-17, 2-18 and 2-19).

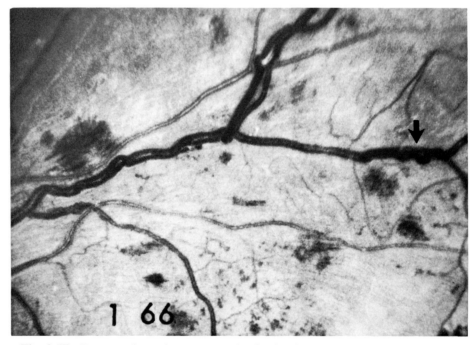

Fig. 2-17. One year later the venous reduplication in Fig. 2-16 has extended proximally. Marked venous beading has developed (arrow) (cf. Figs. 2-15, 2-18 and 2-19).

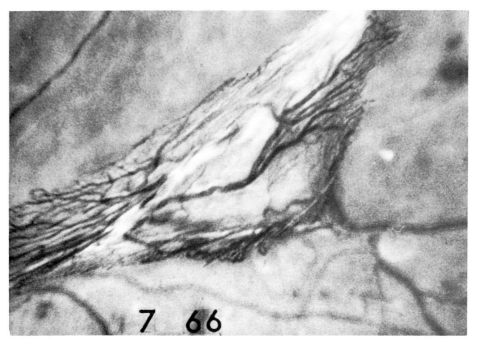

Fig. 2-18. Six months later, a large network of surface new vessels arises from the venous beading of Fig. 2-17 (cf. Figs. 2-15, 2-16 and 2-19).

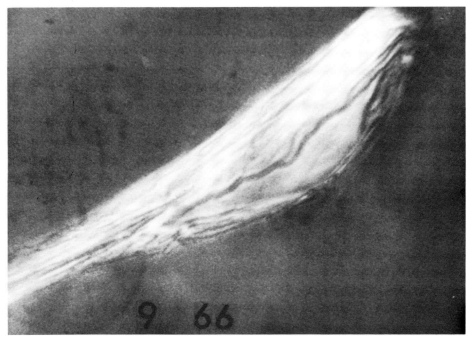

Fig. 2-19. Two months later there is hemorrhage into the space between retina and formed vitreous (cf. Figs. 2-15, 2-16, 2-17 and 2-18).

to appear and break forward through the internal limiting membrane and then to grow on the surface of the retina. First, let us follow the changes that occur in this vein. In Figure 2-16 this vein is double-barrelled above the A/V crossing, but below that the vein still looks relatively normal. In Figure 2-17, 1 year later, the vein is reduplicated back to its junction with the superior temporal vein and appears to be twisted around itself. Further temporally along the superior temporal vein there is marked beading in an area from which new vessels later arose (Fig. 2-18).

The hemorrhages and some of the dilated vessels get "better" between Figures 2-15 & 2-17. I suspect this means that the retina is *more* ischemic and that *more* capillaries have been shut off, and there is perhaps so much ischemia that the vasoproliferative stimulus has stopped; or perhaps the stimulus is there and the endothelial cells are not responding to it. This is highly conjectural, but there is the possibility that this "improvement" is really not improvement. I have the feeling that these eyes go through a stage in which vasoproliferation is very active and then, if the eye is not lost at that point, they go into this stage we call "remission" or "regression" or "burned out," in which I think there are even less patent vessels than there are here.

At any rate, these *intra*retinal changes seem to be getting better, and the *pre*retinal changes are going to begin. Note that where the marked beading is in Figure 2-17, 6 months later (Fig. 2-18) there is a large net of surface new vessels. In Figure 2-18 the retina is slightly out of focus. The reason for this is that the new vessels are slightly anterior to the retina, because the vitreous has begun to contract, pulling the vessels forward. Since the camera is focused on the vessels, the retina behind the vessels is a little out of focus. Shortly after this, vitreous hemorrhage occurred (Fig. 2-19), and another characteristic thing has happened: some of the new vessels have regressed and have been replaced by fibrous tissue. Now the vitreous has not shrunk very much between Figures 2-18 and 2-19, but vitreous hemorrhage has occurred. The hemorrhage is confined to the fluid vitreous behind the detached solid vitreous. I would guess that there is perhaps 1 mm between the plane of the new vessels and the retina. In front of this plane the vitreous remains formed and relatively solid; between the retina and the new vessels is a thin layer of watery fluid vitreous now filled with a suspension of red cells, preventing visualization of the retina.

Fluorescein has been a very valuable tool in looking at diabetic retinopathy. Figure 2-20 is a left eye. There is an obvious wheel of new vessels. Figure 2-21 is a very early stage in the fluorescein angiogram: Choroidal filling has begun, but we can hardly see any fluorescein in the retinal arterioles yet. We see the retinal vessels in silhouette against the choroid. The fluorescein has not gotten to the new vessels yet, but it will shortly. Figure 2-22 is the arterial phase. Fluorescein has filled the arteries and is just barely beginning to fill the new vessels. In Figure 2-23, some 4 to 6 seconds later, already we can see that the fluorescein is being washed out of the arterioles; but notice the marked staining of the arterial wall. The fluorescein has already zipped through the new vessels and some of it has begun to leak out. Note the markedly beaded vein in the lower right part of the figure. Some of the dark areas adjacent to it correspond to hemorrhages which obscure the choroid; but the hemorrhages are not extensive enough to explain *all* of the obscuration of the choroid. The choroid

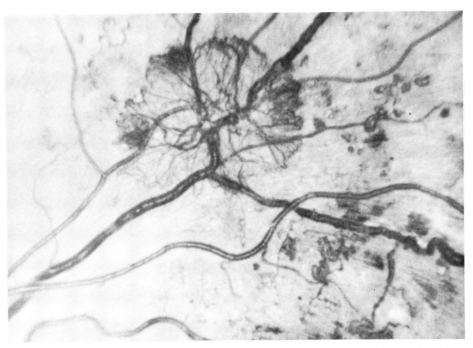

Fig. 2-20. Photograph of new vessel wheel (cf. Figs. 2-21, 2-22, 2-23 and 2-24).

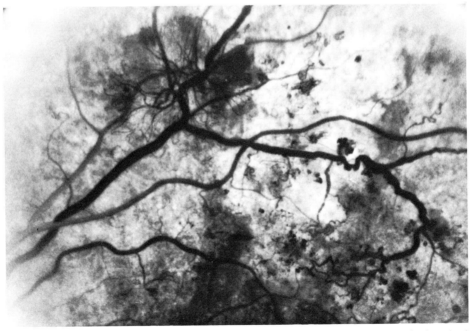

Fig. 2-21. Fluorescein angiogram in choroidal phase. Dye has not reached retinal arterioles (cf. Figs. 2-20, 2-22, 2-23 and 2-24).

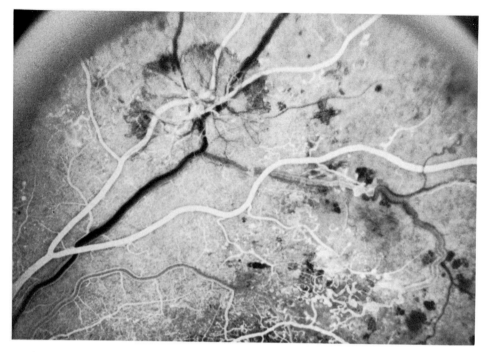

Fig. 2-22. Fluorescein angiogram during arterial phase (cf. Figs. 2-20, 2-21, 2-23 and 2-24).

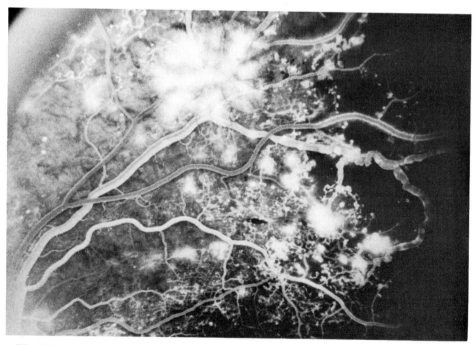

Fig. 2-23. Fluorescein angiogram in venous phase. Note staining of arteriolar walls and leakage from new vessels (cf. Figs. 2-20, 2-21, 2-22 and 2-24).

is obscured, I believe, by very faint soft exudates. This typical fluorescein appearance is often cited as evidence that retinal capillaries are closed. If only the retinal capillaries failed to fill, we would expect the *choroid* to remain visible, but it does not. Actually, the soft exudates are present *because* the retinal capillaries are obliterated, presumably, but there is more to the fluorescein appearance than their closure. Presumably faint soft exudate is more opaque to the fluorescein system than it is to the white light-color system. I certainly agree that there is obliteration of retinal capillaries in an area such as this. In Figure 2-24, several minutes later, we see marked leakage of fluorescein. Fluorescein leakage in diabetic retinopathy occurs both within the retina and in the vitreous, but it is much more profuse in the vitreous. This is a good way to decide whether something is really a new vessel or not. If one gets marked leakage of fluorescein in the late pictures from a little squiggle on the surface of the retina, this usually means the squiggle is a new vessel on the retina rather than a vessel within the retina.

In Figure 2-25, in another patient's left eye (1962), there are a few new vessels on the nerve head and very few elsewhere. About a year later (Fig. 2-26) there has been a little growth of the new vessels, but not much. Figure 2-27, just a month or two later, shows more progression. Six months after this (Fig. 2-28) there has been a marked increase in new vessels. I would like to emphasize that the nature of this disease is to go along with a few new vessels here and there and not do much for perhaps a year or two, and then all of a sudden the patient gets into trouble in a hurry. As you can see, between Figures 2-28 and 2-29 a lot of trouble has occurred. In Figure 2-29 the disc is out of focus down at the bottom of a funnel of detached retina, new vessels, and fibrous tissue, all of which have

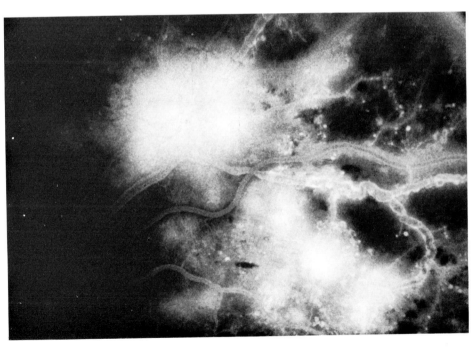

Fig. 2-24. Fluorescein angiogram in late phase. Note leakage within retina is surpassed by new vessel leakage into vitreous (cf. Figs. 2-20, 2-21, 2-22 and 2-23).

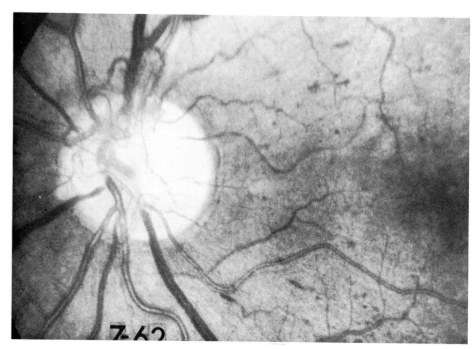

Fig. 2-25. New vessels are mostly limited to the nerve head (cf. Figs. 2-26, 2-27, 2-28 and 2-29).

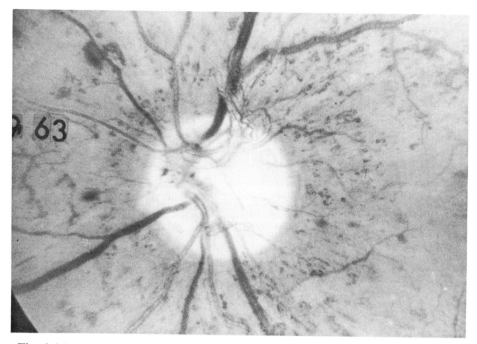

Fig. 2-26. One year later, minimal new vessel growth has occurred (cf. Figs. 2-25, 2-27, 2-28 and 2-29).

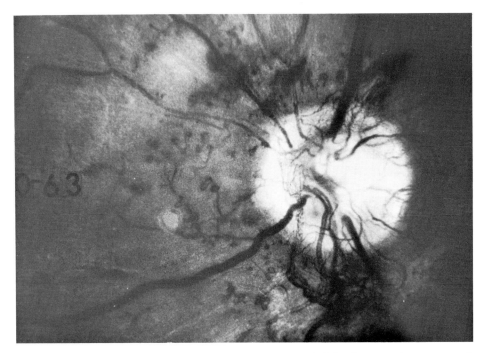

Fig. 2-27. After a few additional weeks, there is a definite increase in new vessels (cf. Figs. 2-25, 2-26, 2-28 and 2-29).

been pulled forward by contraction of the vitreous and of the fibrous tissue itself. The retina is totally detached.

Question from the audience. Had there been vitreous hemorrhage in this eye previously?
Dr. Davis. No, there had not. I think more commonly than not one does see vitreous hemorrhage in eyes like this. I consider the older idea that vitreous hemorrhage is what stimulates the production of fibrous tissue to be erroneous.

Figure 2-30 illustrates the left eye of another juvenile diabetic patient as it appeared in January 1963. There are lots of dot hemorrhages, some linear flame-shaped hemorrhages, and lots of IRMAs. There may be early new vessels on the disc. A couple of months later (Fig. 2-31) the new vessels on the disc are a little more definite. A preretinal hemorrhage has appeared. Two months later (Fig. 2-32) there has been remarkable progression. You can hardly see the disc margins. The new vessels that had begun over the center of the disc are growing extensively across its margins. Two months later (Fig. 2-33) it is difficult to decide, without looking at the next picture (Fig. 2-34), what is happening. After looking at Figure 2-34, it seems clear that improvement had already begun in Figure 2-33. These new vessels are narrower, the retinal changes are perhaps getting a little better, but the improvement is really convincing when you look at Figure 2-34 and see that most of these new vessels have disappeared. The little fibrous plaque and new vessel over the superior temporal vein have stayed about the same through all this, the intraretinal changes have gotten better, the retinal edema has gone

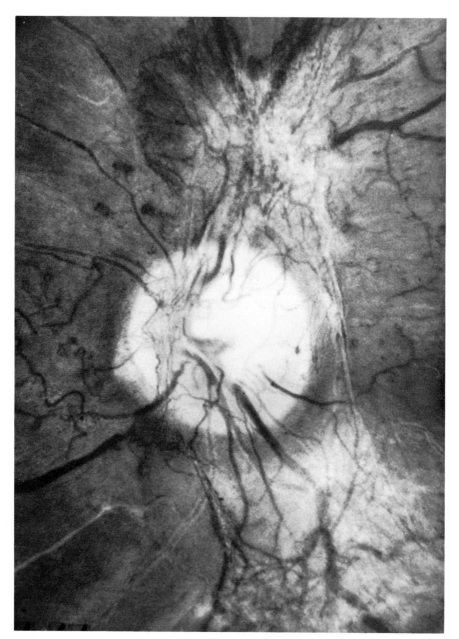

Fig. 2-28. Six months later, there is a marked progression (cf. Figs. 2-25, 2-26, 2-27 and 2-29).

away, leaving hard exudates (edema residues) and most of the new vessels have gone away. Unless I emphasize that this does not happen very often I would be just as guilty by suggesting that this is the typical course, as is sometimes the case when you are shown the results of treatment. I have *selected* a remarkable, dramatic, spontaneous remission, to remind you to be on your guard when someone presents a remarkable, dramatic, "result" of treatment. What we really need are

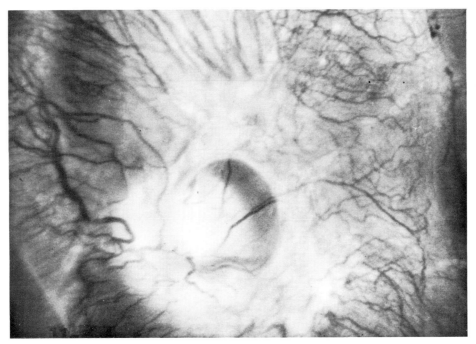

Fig. 2-29. After further progression, a total traction detachment of the retina is present (cf. Figs. 2-25, 2-26, 2-27 and 2-28).

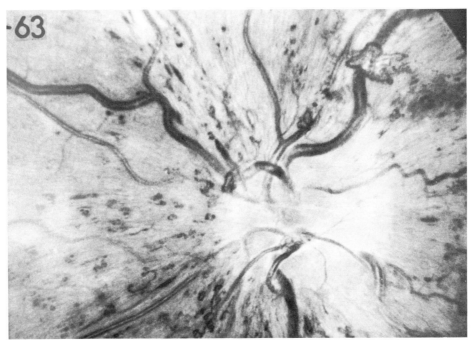

Fig. 2-30. Juvenile diabetic whose nerve head is surrounded by hemorrhage and IRMA's (cf. Figs. 2-31, 2-32, 2-33 and 2-34).

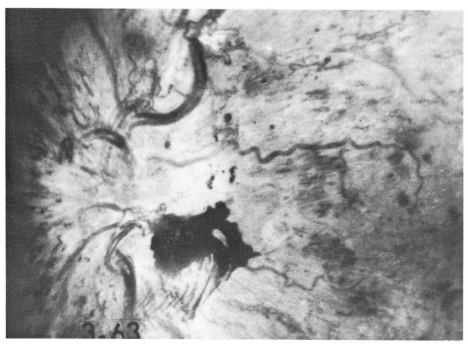

Fig. 2-31. Two months later there are more definite disc new vessels and preretinal hemorrhage has occurred (cf. Figs. 2-30, 2-32, 2-33 and 2-34).

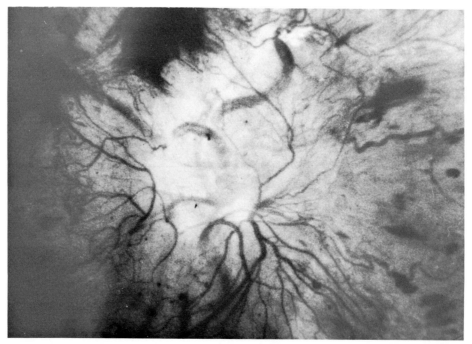

Fig. 2-32. After two more months, new vessels have obscured the disc (cf. Figs. 2-30, 2-31, 2-33 and 2-34).

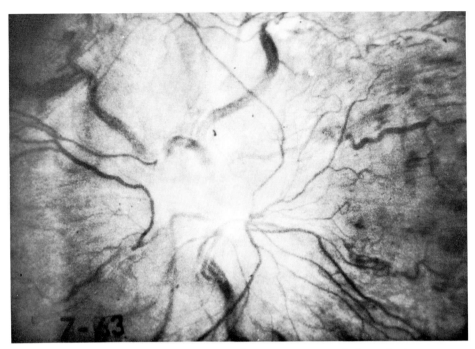

Fig. 2-33. Two months later, new vessels are narrower and the retinal appearance is spontaneously improving (cf. Figs. 2-30, 2-31, 2-32 and 2-34).

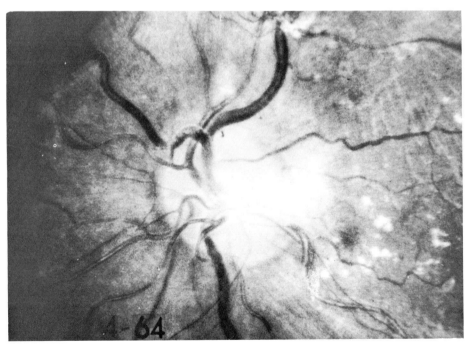

Fig. 2-34. Continued spontaneous improvement has occurred (cf. Figs. 2-30, 2-31, 2-32 and 2-33).

numbers on the screen comparing randomly selected treated and untreated eyes; but we will talk more about that later.

The patient's vision at the end was 20/30. He stayed this way for about 4 years and then began to progress again with regrowth of new vessels, and with vitreous hemorrhage in both eyes. Even though the retinopathy in this patient's right eye, which I have not shown, looked substantially regressed at the beginning, he has now lost useful vision in both eyes. He was a bricklayer, and is no longer able to work. As a matter of fact, he can hardly get around.

I present one more patient—again, highly selected. Figure 2-35 illustrates the right eye of a patient with adult onset diabetes who came in complaining of blurred vision before the diagnosis of diabetes was made. I emphasize that this is an adult onset patient. In the course of the next couple of years, perhaps because his diabetes was controlled (but I am dubious about that), there was remarkable regression of his hemorrhages, hard exudates, etc. (Fig. 2-36). We would certainly think that this represents improvement, but I want to show one other field in this eye. Figure 2-37 is the superior temporal quadrant of the same eye. The appearance is much like Figure 2-35, with hemorrhages, hard exudates, retinal edema, venous beading, and tortuous small vessels that may be IRMA or perhaps new vessels. Two years later, (Fig. 2-38) the intraretinal changes have improved, but here there is no longer any question about the new vessels. They are clearly preretinal. Has the patient gotten better or worse? It's hard to say. Another year later (Fig. 2-39) the new vessels have regressed partially, but there is still fibrous tissue. This patient still has the potential of very easily losing his vision if and when the vitreous and this fibrous tissue contract.

In summary, I should like to remind you of the four processes that I think

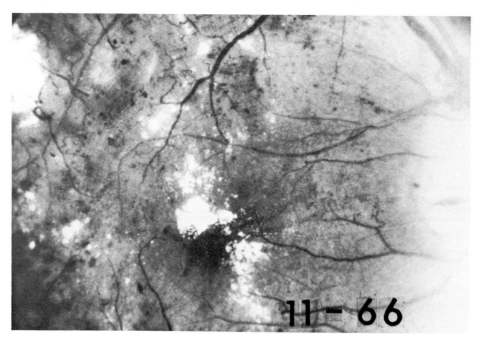

Fig. 2-35. Adult onset diabetic with diabetic retinopathy (cf. Figs. 2-36, 2-37, 2-38 and 2-39).

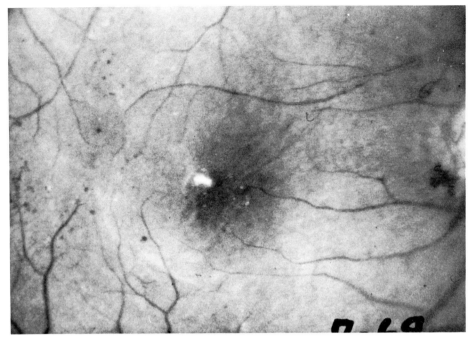

Fig. 2-36. After two and one half years, concurrent with improved diabetic control, there has been a marked improvement in the retinopathy (cf. Figs. 2-35, 2-37, 2-38 and 2-39).

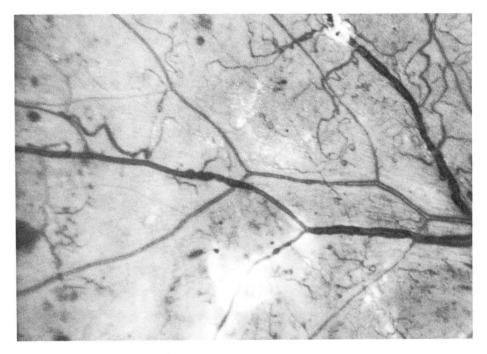

Fig. 2-37. Superior temporal retina at same time as Fig. 2-35. Tortuous small vessels may be IRMA's or new vessels (cf. Figs. 2-35, 2-36, 2-38 and 2-39).

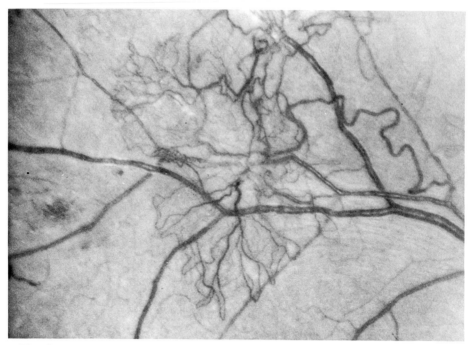

Fig. 2-38. Two and one half years later, the intraretinal changes have improved (cf. Figs. 2-35, 2-36, 2-37 and 2-39).

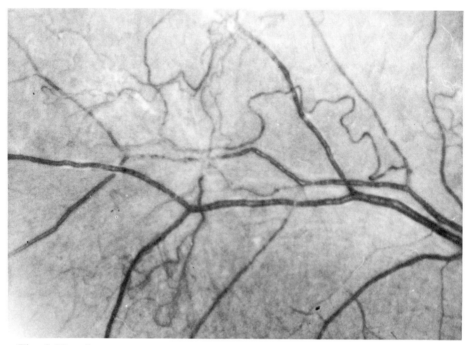

Fig. 2-39. One year later, new vessels have partially regressed (cf. Figs. 2-35, 2-36, 2-37 and 2-38).

are going on in the retina in this disease: (1) obliteration of retinal vessels; (2) proliferation of endothelial cells and fibrous tissue; (3) increased permeability in the vessel walls; and (4) contraction of the fibrous tissue and of the vitreous. I am not as sure as I used to be that it is really the vitreous that is contracting in these patients. Probably there is a thin transparent layer of fibrous tissue that grows along the posterior surface of the vitreous with the new vessels, and it may well be this that is contracting rather than the vitreous itself.

ACKNOWLEDGMENT

Figures 2-4 and 2-11 were supplied through the courtesy of Dr. Ronald Engerman.

REFERENCE

1. Esmann V, Lundbaek K, Madsen PM: Acta Med Scand 174:378–384, 1963
   Types of exudates in diabetic retinopathy.

Francis I. Caird

Chapter 3
Epidemiology of Diabetic Retinopathy

Epidemiologic data can be used in two ways with regard to a topic such as diabetic retinopathy. They can be used to define and describe the size of the problem, and also to throw light on possible etiologic factors. Both of these approaches can be made in the case of diabetic retinopathy, and in both instances yield interesting and important facts and conclusions.

The size of the problem posed by diabetic retinopathy is best illustrated by its contribution to blindness. The most satisfactory and complete data are those for the United Kingdom from 1955 to 1962,[9] which were amplified by the British Diabetic Association's Committee on Blindness.[3] In England and Wales in the years 1955 to 1962, an average of 670 people were registered as blind each year because of diabetic retinopathy (Fig. 3-1). This was from a population of approximately 50 million. Three-quarters of these people were women, although under the age of 50 there is a considerable excess of men. Ninety-two percent of people who are registered blind because of diabetic retinopathy are over 50, and nearly half are over 70, at the time of registration. This puts into perspective the idea that diabetic retinopathy is a problem of young people. It is not. Blindness, at least, is a problem of later middle and old age. During the 7 years from 1955 to 1962 there was no substantial change in the annual incidence of blindness due to diabetic retinopathy, but since then, there has been an increase of the order of approximately 30 to 50 percent, which is shown in both the figures for England and Wales and in separately collected figures for the West of Scotland.[3] This is presumed to reflect a true increase in incidence, rather than an increase in the tendency of diabetics to take advantage of the benefits derived from registration. A further increase above the figure shown in Figure 3-1 is also necessary because there is good evidence that those with visual impairment sufficient to qualify them for registration as blind may not in fact do so.[5] This failure to register applies in particular to elderly women who are nondiabetic, as well as to elderly women who are diabetic. The Committee on Blindness concluded that the figures shown in Figure 3-1 now represent about half the true incidence.

The importance of retinopathy as a cause of blindness is shown in Figure 3-2.

Average No. of New Blind Registrations per year attributed to Diabetic Retinopathy

(England and Wales 1955–62; after Sorsby 1966)

Age	15–29	30–49	50–9	60–9	70+	Total
Males	3	28	26	48	48	153
Females	2	18	60	188	250	518
Total	5	46	86	236	298	671

Fig. 3-1. Average number of new blind registrations per year attributed to diabetic retinopathy in England and Wales, 1955 to 1962. (Adapted with permission from Sorsby A: Rep Public Health & Med Subjects 114, London, HMSO, 1966).

In 10 percent of blind registrations in middle-aged men, and in 20 percent in middle-aged women, blindness is due to diabetic retinopathy. The figure for all ages and both sexes is about 7 percent. These proportions also require upward revision, especially probably in middle age. But as they stand, they show that in England and Wales, at least, diabetic retinopathy is the fifth commonest cause of blindness at all ages taken together, being exceeded by senile macular lesions, cataract, glaucoma, and, narrowly, by myopic chorioretinal atrophy. Data from other countries are essentially comparable. What differences there are can be attributed with fair confidence to differences in registration procedures and differences in the prevalence of diabetes itself. Thus, in Denmark, diabetic retinopathy is the cause of over 20 percent of all registrations, and not 7 percent as in the United Kingdom.[10] But in Denmark, few people over 70, and none under 30, register under the scheme in question, so that the higher proportion thus reflects

Percentage of New Blind Registrations attributed

to Diabetic Retinopathy (from Sorsby, 1966)

Age	15–29	30–49	50–9	60–9	70+	All Ages
Males	4	11	10	9	2	4.4
Females	4	10	19	21	5	8.6

Fig. 3-2. Percentage of new blind registrations attributed to diabetic retinopathy in England and Wales, 1955 to 1962. (Adapted with permission from Sorsby A: Rep Public Health & Med Subjects 114, London, HMSO, 1966).

the situation in middle age, where 10 to 20 percent is a very fair figure (Fig. 3-2). Diabetic retinopathy does not figure as a cause of blindness in Iceland, where diabetes is very rare; but it is a major cause of blindness in Malta, where diabetes is very common.[2] I have no doubt the Pima Indians will come out even worse.

The pattern of prevalence of blindness from diabetic retinopathy can be inferred from that of incidence. The Committee on Blindness[3] concluded that the true prevalence in England and Wales is of the order of 100 per million of all ages. It is possible to calculate that about 2 percent of the total diabetic population is blind, a figure that is 10 times that for the general population. So, the diabetic is at least 10 times, and probably nearer 20 times, more likely to become blind from retinopathy than a nondiabetic from all the other causes of blindness put together.[3] This is perhaps the most striking and possibly, therefore, the best measure of the importance of diabetic retinopathy.

This is the contribution of epidemiologic methods to the assessment of the size of the problem presented by diabetic retinopathy. The contribution of these methods to understanding the etiology of retinopathy is also considerable. It is perhaps pertinent to remark at this point that the facts of epidemiology are facts, and they are not to be discounted because they do not emerge from a laboratory or from animal experiments. Indeed, they need to be taken into account in any comprehensive hypothesis about the cause of diabetic microvascular disease. The most useful question to ask is, What diabetics develop retinopathy? Figure 3-3 shows the frequency of clinically diagnosed retinopathy in relation to age and sex in some 4000 observations on 2000 adult diabetics who attended the Diabetic

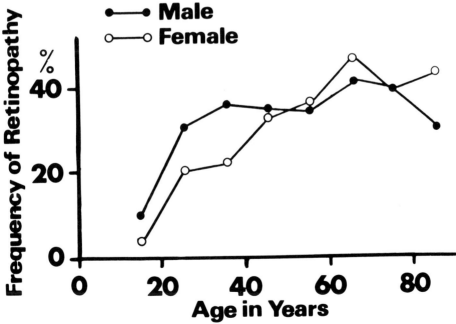

Fig. 3-3. Frequency of diabetic retinopathy by age and sex. (Reprinted with permission from Caird FI, Pirie A, Ramsell TG: Diabetes and the Eye. Oxford, Blackwell, 1969).

Clinic in Oxford, England.[2] There are no observations in children, but other observations have shown convincingly that clinically detectable retinopathy is virtually unknown under the age of 10, and very rare under the age of 15. Over that age it increases steadily in frequency up to the age of about 40 or so; it then remains roughly constant at around 30 to 35 percent. The frequency in men and women is the same over age of 40; but, as with blindness, there is an excess of men with retinopathy under that age, which is technically significant in the 35-to-39-age group. This parallel with the situation among the diabetic blind is unexplained and interesting. More illuminating is the prevalence of retinopathy in relation to age at diagnosis and duration of diabetes. Figure 3-4 shows the frequency of retinopathy at the time of diagnosis of diabetes.[8] Retinopathy is rare under the age of 40 at the time of diagnosis, but over that age it increases steadily to reach a frequency of about 10 percent. It is possible to calculate that this prevalence of retinopathy in older diabetics could be accounted for by an average duration of diabetes before diagnosis of no more than about 2 years—a figure which is in reasonable agreement with the duration of symptoms of diabetes that people in this age group often admit to. The frequently made suggestion that those people who have retinopathy at diagnosis must have had true diabetes for 10, 15, or even 20 years, is in error. The pattern in relation to duration of diabetes is shown in Figure 3-5.[1] This is typical of several comparable studies. In those whose diabetes is diagnosed before the age of 30, retinopathy is relatively unusual until after 5 years of diabetes have gone by, but thereafter, the frequency rises rapidly to reach 50 percent at about 12 years, and 75 percent or more after 20 years. Others have mentioned an eventual prevalence of 100 percent, but this appears to be derived from projection rather than from actual observation. When diabetes develops in middle age—between 30 and 59—the frequency within 5 years is rather higher, but the increase in frequency with increasing duration occurs steadily, up to approximately the same eventual frequency of about 80 percent. Over the age of 60 at diagnosis there is a still higher starting point and a slower rise. For practical purposes it is simple to remember that after

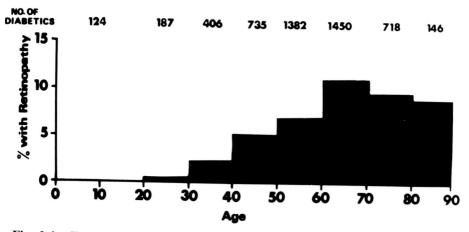

Fig. 3-4. Frequency of diabetic retinopathy at diagnosis of diabetes, by age. (Reprinted with permission from Soler NG, Fitzgerald MG, Malins J, Summer ROC: Br Med J 3:567, 1969).

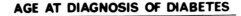

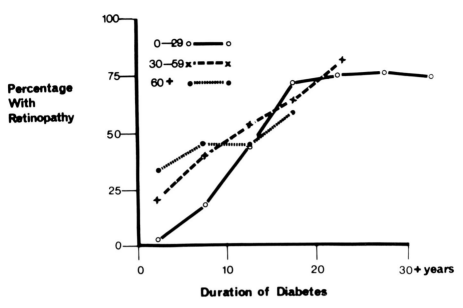

Fig. 3-5. Frequency of retinopathy by age at diagnosis and duration of diabetes. (Reprinted with permission from Burditt AF, Caird FI, Draper GJ: Q J Med 37:303, 1968).

10 to 15 years of diabetes, diabetics of all ages at diagnosis have about a 50-percent chance of having retinopathy.

There are many difficulties in the classification of retinopathy, but if the term "malignant" retinopathy is used instead of "proliferative," [1] Figure 3-6 shows the frequency of malignant retinopathy in relation to duration of diabetes.[6] In diabetics under the age of 30 at diagnosis, malignant retinopathy is rare until 15 years of diabetes have passed. Even over that duration it is only found in about 10 percent of diabetics. The only discordant line is that from the Joslin Clinic,[11] and it is possible, though not certain, that this represents differing definitions, observer variation, and possibly also that diabetics with visual symptoms due to malignant retinopathy may attend the Joslin Clinic more often than those who do not have visual problems. Certainly in Oxford a prevalence of around 10 percent after 15 to 20 years would seem to be accurate.

There is no definite evidence of any particular racial susceptibility to diabetic retinopathy outside the known racial and ethnic variation in the frequency of diabetes itself. The literature is extremely confusing; much of it totally fails to take into account the dominant importance of age at diagnosis and duration of diabetes. Nor is there, so far as I am aware, any convincing evidence of any familial factor involved in retinopathy itself, which is a different problem from the hereditary background of diabetes. A study of 75 families, each with more than one diabetic member, entirely failed to show any aggregation of patients with retinopathy within families.[2] The question of the frequency of retinopathy in diabetes of known cause is of great theoretical, although little practical, importance. Figure 3-7 shows the individual cases of clinical retinopathy in secondary diabetes

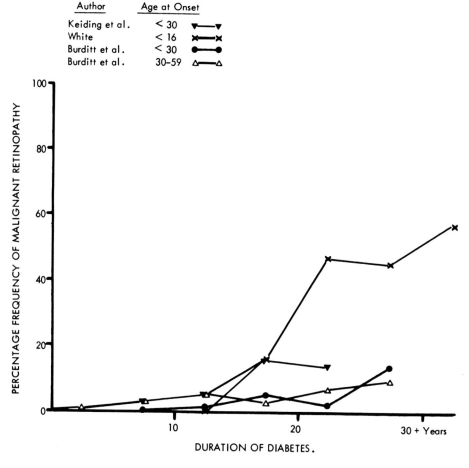

Fig. 3-6. Frequency of "malignant" retinopathy by duration of diabetes.

in man reported up to 1969;[2] since then there have been 9 more cases reported in the diabetes of hemachromatosis.[4] In no instance is the number of cases reported large. The most important single point is that the duration of known diabetes at the time of detection of retinopathy is almost always over 5 years, and very often over 10 years. This is much the same as in diabetes of known cause.

Finally, it is important to remember that diabetic retinopathy is only part of a generalized disorder of blood vessels, and that it is therefore a condition with a mortality. A life table analysis of the mortality of four groups of diabetics matched for age and sex, but having different degrees of retinopathy (Fig. 3-8), shows that if the fundi were normal or only microaneurysms were present, then mortality is only slightly different. But if more advanced retinopathy is present, and particularly if malignant retinopathy, with new vessel formation, proliferative changes, or preretinal hemorrhage is present, then there is a substantial mortality over a period of 5 to 7 years. This is even more clearly shown by the mortality of the diabetic blind, whose death rate is about 14 to 15 percent per year at all ages (Fig. 3-9).[7] It is very interesting that a small study carried out in the west of Scotland[3]

CLINICAL RETINOPATHY IN SECONDARY
DIABETES IN MAN

Cause of Diabetes	No. of Cases Reported	Duration of Diabetes at Detection of Retinopathy (Years)
Chronic Pancreatitis	7	9, 9, 12, 13, 16, 18, 24.
Pancreatectomy	2	3, 11.
Haemochromatosis	10	2, 7, 8, >8, >8, >8, 11, 13, 15, >15, >15.
Cushing's Syndrome	2	9, 11.
Acromegaly	3	2, 8, ?10.
Phaeochromocytoma	0	–

Fig. 3-7. Clinical retinopathy in secondary diabetes in man. (Reprinted with permission from Caird FI, Pirie A, Ramsell TG: Diabetes and the Eye. Oxford, Blackwell 1969).

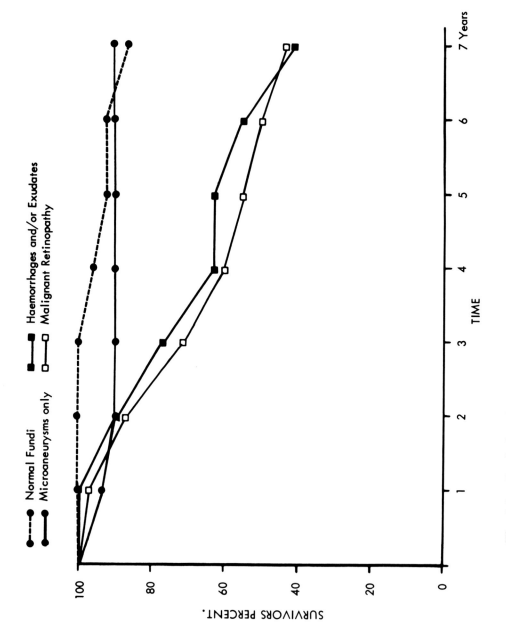

Fig. 3-8. Survival and severity of retinopathy. (Reprinted with permission from Caird FI, Pirie A, Ramsell TG: Diabetes and the Eye. Oxford, Blackwell, 1969).

42

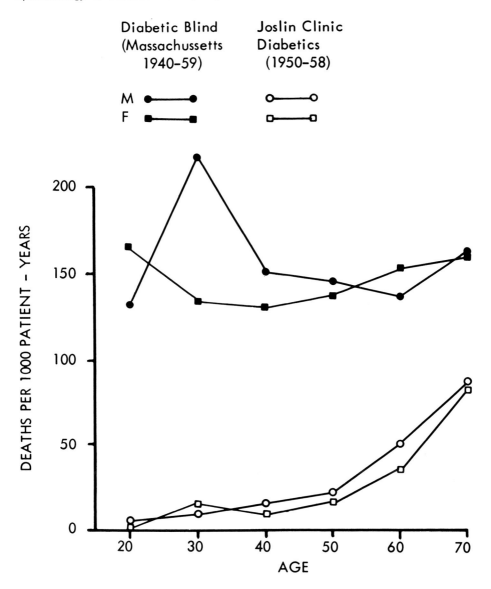

Fig. 3-9. Survival of the diabetic blind. (Reprinted with permission from Rogot E: US Public Health Rep 80:1025, 1965).

showed an exactly similar mortality of 14 percent per year, a good example of the fact that diabetics from all over the world resemble each other very closely. The mortality of the diabetic blind in the younger ages is of the order of 20 times that of all diabetics of the same age (Fig. 3-9). Even at the age of 70, the excess is of the order of twofold. This high mortality is due to concomitant diabetic renal disease and coronary artery disease. But even a mortality of 14 to 15 percent per year means that the mean survival of the diabetic blind is of the order of 3 to 3.5 years, and that as many as 20 percent are still alive 10 years after registration as blind. The problems of rehabilitation, management, and support that this figure represents bear thinking about by physicians and ophthalmologists alike.

REFERENCES

1. Burditt AF, Caird FI, Draper GJ: The natural history of diabetic retinopathy. Q J M 37:303, 1968
2. Caird FI, Pirie A, Ramsell TG: Diabetes and the Eye. Oxford, Blackwell, 1969
3. Committee on Blindness: Report on Diabetic Blindness in the United Kingdom. London, British Diabetic Association, 1970
4. Dymock IW, Williams R: Haemachromatosis and diabetes. Postgrad Med J 47:79, 1971
5. Graham, PA, Wallace J, Welsby E, Grace HJ: Evaluation of postal detection of registrable blindness. Br J Prev Soc Med 22:238, 1968
6. Keiding NR, Root HF, Marble A: Importance of control of diabetes in prevention of vascular complications. JAMA 150:964, 1952
7. Rogot E: Note on mortality among the diabetic blind. US Public Health Rep 80:1025, 1965
8. Soler NG, Fitzgerald MG, Malins J, Summers ROC: Retinopathy at diagnosis of diabetes, with special reference to patients under 40 years of age. Br Med J 3:567, 1969
9. Sorsby A: The incidence and cause of blindness in England and Wales 1948-62. Rept Public Health & Med Subjects 114, London, HMSO 1966
10. Vedel-Jensen N: The causes of blindness in 1000 consecutive new members of the Danish Society for the Blind. Dan Med Bull 9:185, 1962
11. White P: Childhood diabetes. Diabetes 9: 345, 1960

Question. How can we ascribe diabetes mellitus to a primary vascular disease if secondary causes of hyperglycemia will produce retinopathy typical of diabetes? **Dr. Siperstein.** All studies that have attempted to determine the prevalence of diabetic retinopathy, of renal disease, typical intercapillary glomerulosclerosis in patients with pancreatitis, pheochromocytoma or Cushing's disease have reported, with one exception—that of Becker and Miller—a remarkedly low prevalence rate. Every other study would say the prevalence of diabetic microangiopathy in secondary diabetes is no greater than the prevalence of genetic diabetes in the general population. We have in fact used these data to support the contention that the hyperglycemia per se, in the absence of genetic diabetes mellitus, does not produce microangiopathy even though the hyperglycemia has been present for 15 or 20 years. **Dr. Kohner.** We consider their glucose tolerance abnormal if the fasting blood sugar is over 110. We would also consider it abnormal if the 2-hour blood sugar was over 200. I do not think that diabetes is purely an abnormality of glucose tolerance. I think that one very important point was left out and that is the question of insulin. It is the glucose-insulin ratio that matters. What is the insulin response to a glucose load? And we have not heard it either from Dr. Davis or from Dr. Siperstein. I would also like to make the point that maybe a high blood sugar does not matter all that much if you look at microangiopathy, but I would like to point out that it does matter as far as the patient's prognosis for life is concerned, because it has been shown by the Scandanavian group, without any doubt, that high blood sugar is related to arterial disease. And what do these patients die from? They die from coronary artery disease, from renal disease, and from cerebral vascular disease. So, yes, I do think we should treat patients who have high blood sugars. I do think we should treat some of this damage—not with tablets and not with insulin, unless they have symptoms which require it. But diabetic dietary treatment is important if we want to keep these patients alive. We do not necessarily tell our patients that they have diabetes, but we do tell them they have a carbohydrate intolerance because it is our duty to tell them so. I think it is very unfortunate that the patient gets adverse insurance or that he is grounded if he is a pilot. I certainly do not think that diabetes requiring tablet treatment, or diet treatment only, should ground the pilot. But that is the social system which would be ordered for that and not your diagnosis. Your duty as a physician is to keep your patients alive and keep them healthy.

Dr. Siperstein. I can hardly disagree with your last statement regarding morality and the duty of the physician. I would only disagree, on the basis of well-published data, with the definition of an abnormal glucose tolerance test. Please do not blur the distinction between a high glucose tolerance test and fasting hyperglycemia. Unless one wishes to say that 30 to 50 percent of the population requires therapy for diabetes, then one is going to overdiagnose diabetes. Microangiopathy, life expectancy or any other indication of diabetes is poorly correlated with glucose tolerance if proper controls are carried out. There are numerous papers in the literature claiming that there is a relationship between coronary artery disease, cancer, gyngivitis, and glucose intolerance. As I have tried to emphasize, these are based on uncontrolled studies, and the easiest way to prove this is simply to do glucose tolerance tests on patients who have any nonspecific disease. I am just asking you to be cautious in the overdiagnosis of diabetes. The difference in the definition of glucose intolerance in Europe and in the United States in part, I am sure, depend upon different loads of glucose administered—50 g in Europe versus 100 g in the United States—and differences in plasma and blood values. I know of no data that would support the figures of a statistically abnormal glucose intolerance at anything less than 220 at 2 hours. I think this is a difference in fact; the rest is a difference of opinion and methods of administering glucose tolerance tests.

Question from audience. But don't all diabetics have abnormal glucose tolerance tests before they have hyperglycemia?

Dr. Siperstein. That is an excellent question. All overt diabetics go through a period of glucose intolerance, no question about it. But it does not follow a priori that all patients with glucose intolerance become diabetic. It is that logical fallacy that has unfortunately confused people in the field much too long. Let me use an analogy. Almost all patients with cancer lose weight. But most people who lose weight do not have cancer. The problem with the glucose tolerance test is that it is so remarkably nonspecific. Just as weight loss is a poor way of diagnosing cancer, so glucose tolerance is a poor way of diagnosing diabetes.

Chemical diabetes is defined as a normal fasting blood sugar with a decrease in glucose tolerance generally accepted as the Fajans and Conn criteria of 160 blood sugar at 1 hour, 120 at 2 hours; plasma sugars of 185 and 150. Overt diabetes is defined as fasting hyperglycemia. In other words, we will not make the diagnosis of chemical diabetes ever. We consider it a mystical concept that cannot be defined since most patients who bear this diagnosis do not have overt diabetes and never develop it. Again, we only tell a patient he has diabetes when he has proven overt diabetes, i.e., fasting hyperglycemia.

Morton F. Goldberg

Chapter 4

The Role of Ischemia in the Production
of Vascular Retinopathies

In this presentation I would like to present a particular point of view; namely, that ischemia plays a fundamental role in the pathogenesis of proliferative retinopathies in a *variety* of diseases, including diabetic retinopathy. Because diabetic retinopathy in its advanced stages presents a very complicated fundus picture, it is useful to study other diseases which show proliferative changes in the retina, since in many cases the course of events is relatively easier to decipher. It is hoped that the conclusions reached from a study of these diseases might be applicable to a better understanding of the diabetic process in the retina. Consequently, I would like to discuss several systemic diseases characterized by proliferative changes in the retina, all of which have, as an underlying pathogenetic factor, a significant ischemic process in the retina.

SICKLE CELL ANEMIA

The retinal ischemic process in sickling is apparently induced by microemboli or viscosity-induced thrombosis in the retinal vasculature. Normal red blood cells have a biconcave-disc shape, but sickled red blood cells adopt a very characteristic sickle-shaped configuration. Not only is the configuration abnormal, but also these cells are rather rigid, unlike the normal, pliable red cells. Consequently, it is very easy for these abnormal cells to impact in small retinal blood vessels, as well as elsewhere in the body; ischemia and hypoxia are the results. In the retina of patients with certain forms of sickling there is a temporal predilection for the occluded arterioles and capillary bed and also a far peripheral predilection (between the equator of the eye and the ora serrata). In these respects the ischemic process in sickling is somewhat different from that in diabetes, but it is not altogether different.

Upon examination of the retina, one can see that there are abrupt arteriolar occlusions in sickling (Fig. 4-1). One may observe ophthalmoscopically a typical "silver wire," in which fluorescein angiography confirms the absence of perfusion. A distinct border can be observed between the posteriorly (centrally) perfused retina and the anteriorly (peripherally) nonperfused retina at about the equatorial plane

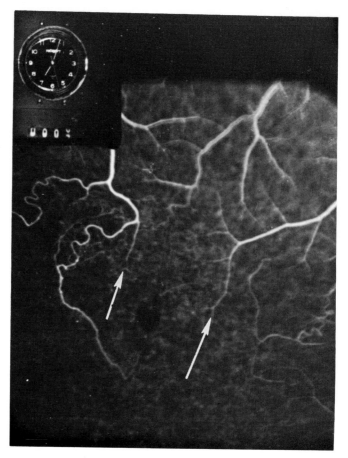

Fig. 4-1. Retinal vascular occlusions (*arrows*) in sickle thalassemia (Reprinted with permission from Goldberg MF et al.: Arch Intern Med 128:33, 1971).

(Fig. 4-2). In fact, the entire peripheral retina is often completely nonperfused, whereas the posterior retina is generally perfused in a relatively normal fashion. Occasionally, macular vessels may be occluded also.

Trypsin digestion studies confirm these angiographic and ophthalmoscopic observations. Some of the changes are very similar to those of diabetic retinopathy. For example, the capillary bed may be almost completely acellular (Fig. 4-3) representing poor perfusion and presumed infarction of the capillary bed (Fig. 4-4).

The next stage of proliferative sickle retinopathy that can be observed with a combination of ophthalmoscopy and fluorescein angiography is that of arteriolo-venular anastomoses occurring at the sites of previous arteriolar obstructions. You may translate the term "arteriolo-venular anastomosis" into "shunt vessel" or IRMA (i.e., intraretinal microvascular abnormality), as used in the diabetic, since these vessels appear to arise in a similar fashion. Trypsin studies of sickled retinas show dilated connections between adjacent arterioles and venules; the surrounding capillary bed is completely missing.

The next stage that can be visualized by ophthalmoscopy or fluorescein angiography is the stage of actual neovascular proliferation (Figs. 4-5 and 4-6). These

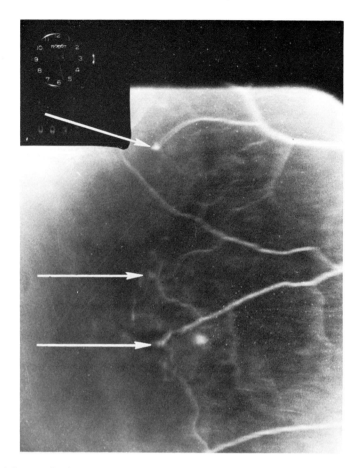

Fig. 4-2. Retinal vascular occlusions (*arrows*) in sickling. Note abrupt equ*atorial* transition zone between perfused retina (*on right*) and nonperfused retina (*on left*). (Reprinted with permission from Goldberg MF et al.: Arch Intern Med 123:33, 1971).

lesions invariably arise at the sites of previous arteriolar occlusions and arteriolovenular anastomoses, and almost invariably grow into the ischemic zone; that is, they grow toward the ora serrata in a very typical fanshaped configuration (Fig. 4-7). These fanshaped proliferations often have aneurysmal dilatations at their growing edge. One might conclude, in a conjectural way perhaps, that this neovascular tissue is growing in a reparative effort, or that it is responding to some stimulus generated by the hypoxic retinal tissue. Vascular proliferation characterizes two major forms of sickling: sickle cell hemoglobin C disease and sickle thalassemia.

Routine histology confirms the fact that there is neovascular tissue growing into the vitreous cavity and that the blood vessels are attached to the posterior hyaloid face. The particular section in Figure 4-8 comes from a patient with sickling, although it might well be in an individual with diabetic retinopathy, retrolental fibroplasia, or any one of a number of proliferative vascular retinopathies. It is of interest to note that these fanshaped configurations have a temporal predilection; in fact, the most commonly involved quadrant is the supratemporal one,

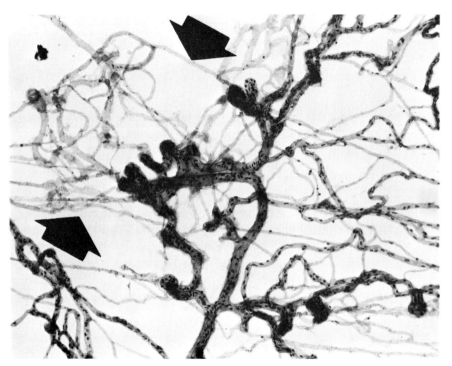

Fig. 4-3. Trypsin digest preparation of retina in sickling. Note acellular capillaries (arrows), which presumably represent absent or poor perfusion. (Reprinted with permission from Romayananda N, Goldberg MF, Green WR: Trans Am Acad Ophthalmol Otolaryngol 77:IP-652–OP-677, 1973).

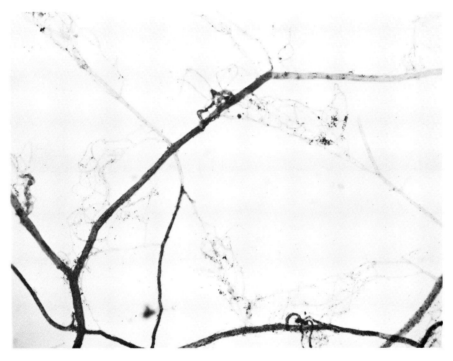

Fig. 4-4. Marked loss of capillary bed in trypsin digested preparation of human retina in sickling.

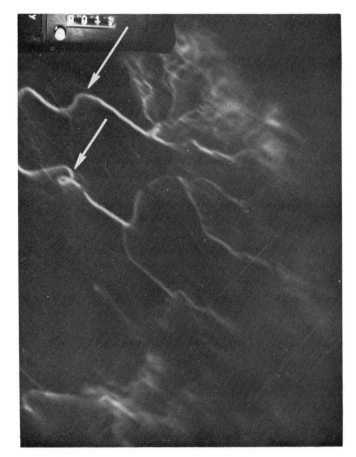

Fig. 4-5. Arteriolar phase of fluorescein angiogram demonstrating retinal neovascularization in sickling. *Arrows* are placed similarly in Figure 4-6 (Reprinted with permission from Goldberg MF et al.: Arch Intern Med 128:33, 1971).

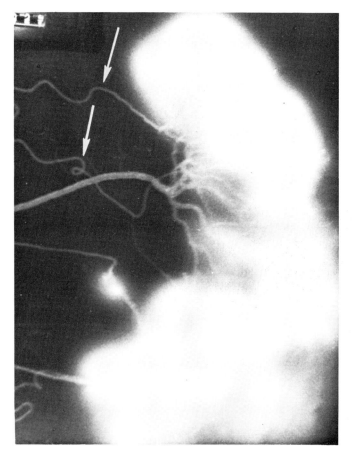

Fig. 4-6. Venous phase of angiogram demonstrating fanshaped configuration of neovascular tissue in sickling. *Arrows* are placed similarly in Figure 4-5 (Reprinted with permission from Goldberg MF et al.: Arch Intern Med 128:33, 1971).

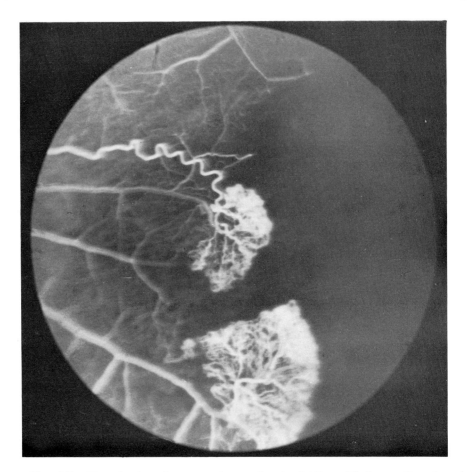

Fig. 4-7. Two fanshaped neovascular patches in sickling. Their growth pattern is in the direction of nonperfused, ischemic retina.

followed by the infratemporal one, followed, in turn, by the supranasal one, and least commonly affected of all is the infranasal quadrant. You will recall that this quadrantic predilection is identical to that observed in proliferative diabetic retinopathy and is very similar to that observed in retrolental fibroplasia.

The next stage that is observable by ophthalmoscopic techniques is spontaneous vitreous hemorrhage emanating from the neovascular tissue. These hemorrhages may be small or massive. They generally arise from the small patch of neovascular tissue which itself is often obscured by the hemorrhage. If one is able to observe the neovascular tissue responsible for the hemorrhage, even in the stage of active hemorrhaging, such a lesion is often amenable to photocoagulation therapy.

Finally, as a consequence of vitreous collapse, traction, and retinal hole formation (possibly exacerbated by the previous stage of vitreous hemorrhage), retinal detachment occurs.

To summarize the state of knowledge in the development of proliferative sickle retinopathy, it is reasonable to conclude that the semiarbitrary classification noted above does seem to describe accurately a spontaneous and naturally occurring

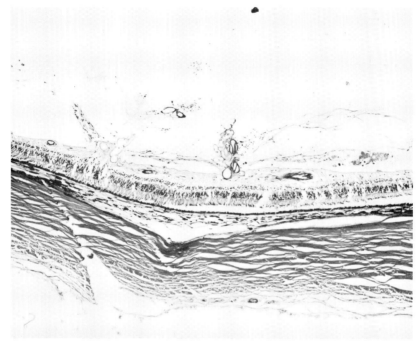

Fig. 4-8. Histologic cross-section of sickled retina shows intravitreal growth of neovascular tissue with attached vitreous strands (Reprinted with permission from Romayananda N, Goldberg MF, Green WR: Trans Am Acad Ophthalmol Otolaryngol 77:OP-652–OP-676, 1973).

sequence of events that is initiated by arteriolar occlusions and ischemia. The following stages of anastomoses, proliferations, hemorrhages, and detachments develop naturally, occurring over either months or years. It would appear that the same sequence of events, with only mild modifications, can be utilized for an understanding and classification of the course of events in other proliferative retinopathies.

RETROLENTAL FIBROPLASIA

In the case of retrolental fibroplasia (RLF), the process leading to arteriolar occlusions is obviously different from that in sickle cell anemia. We will not dwell on the pathogenesis of oxygen toxicity in this disease, but it is necessary to emphasize that the first significant change that is clinically observable in RLF is peripheral arteriolar shutdown and retinal ischemia. For the most part, this occurs in the temporal periphery of the fundus, although other portions are not immune. Subsequently, neovascular proliferations grow, once again in a manner that is seemingly identical to that in sickle cell diseases, into the ischemic zone, that is, towards the ora serrata. It is the subsequent hemorrhaging and fibrosis that lead to dragging of the disc and retina, membrane formation, retinal detachment, and the intravitreal fibrous sheets and bands that give rise to the term retrolental fibroplasia.

Fluorescein angiography (and simple indirect ophthalmoscopy) reveals many similarities between the peripheral neovascularization in RLF and that in the sickling process. There is temporal ischemia and a growing edge of granulation tissue on the surface of the retina. Fluorescein angiography reveals, as in sickling, an abrupt interface between anterior, nonperfused retina and posterior, perfused retina. At the interface, active growth of neovascular tissue occurs. Ultimately, one is left with a stage of fibroplasia and scar tissue formation. Often in this stage, one may be forgetful of the fact that this severe complication is the end result of what is basically an ischemic retinopathy that has induced retinal neovascularization.

OTHER RETINOPATHIES

Proliferative retinopathy also occurs in sarcoidosis. Here, the ischemic process appears to be related to an inflammation in the vascular walls with subsequent thrombosis. Again, fanshaped arteriolovenular malformations can develop. With fluorescein angiography, these AV fans are seen to have an active growing zone, characterized by the leaking of fluorescein. This zone grows into an area of retinal ischemia (Figs. 4-9, 4-10, and 4-11). In retinal sarcoidosis, therefore, one can note once again marked peripheral retinal ischemia, arteriolar obstructions, a

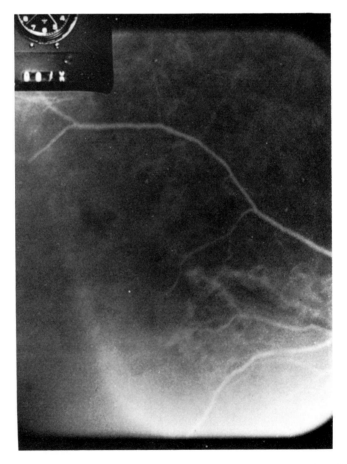

Fig. 4-9. Arterial phase of angiography in sarcoidosis. Fanshaped neovascular capillary bed (*lower right*) is growing toward ischemic zone of retina (*lower left*).

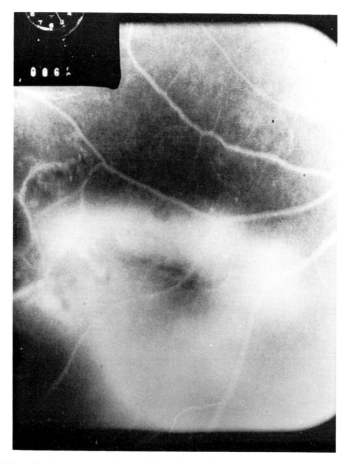

Fig. 4-10. Early venous phase of angiography in sarcoidosis. Marked transudation of dye into the vitreous has occurred (cf. Fig. 4-9).

fanshaped configuration of neovascular tissue growing towards the ischemic zone, and, of course, as in all proliferative retinopathies, there is marked leakage of fluorescein into the vitreous. The same general conclusions can be applied to other proliferative retinopathies reported in the literature, for example, radiation retinitis and leukemic retinopathy. Fluorescein angiography in chronic myelogenous leukemia shows similar characteristics to those observed in sickle cell anemia, retrolental fibroplasia, and sarcoidosis.

The same general characteristics are true of another disease as well. It is uncommonly observed in the United States, but is relatively more common in the Orient, particularly in young females, namely, Takayasu's or pulseless disease. Because of poor vascular perfusion (created by occlusive phenomena in the aorta and in the large arteries of the neck), one finds retinal ischemia developing for 360 degrees and occurring very close to the disc itself. Subsequently, peripapillary neovascularization develops at the interface of perfused and nonperfused retina. The typical ophthalmoscopic feature of pulseless disease therefore, is a peripapillary wreath of anastomotic and proliferative neovascular tissue.

A similar appearance characterizes branch vein occlusion and occasionally

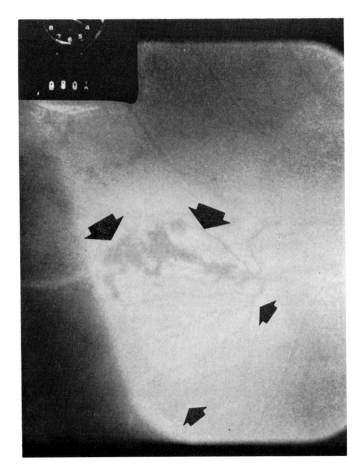

Fig. 4-11. Late venous phase of angiography in sarcoidosis. Neovascular channels appear as dark, linear shadows (*arrows*) surrounded by white intravitreal fluorescein (cf. Figs. 4-9 and 4-10).

central vein occlusion in the retina. Here, again, there has been a tremendously significant ischemic process going on in the retina, presumably from stagnation initiated by the thrombotic process in the branch or central vein. At the interface of the perfused and nonperfused retinal areas, there is once again the potential for the development of neovascular tissue.

DIABETIC RETINOPATHY

What conclusions can we draw with relationship to the diabetic retinopathic process? First of all, there is considerable evidence that ischemia once again plays a fundamental role in the pathogenesis of all aspects of diabetic retinopathy, including the proliferative ones. Eva Kohner [1] was one of the first investigators to show that scotomas in the visual fields of diabetic patients were frequent, even if observable retinopathy was not apparent. In one particular series, 50 percent of diabetics without ophthalmoscopically observable retinopathy had small scotomas demonstrated in their visual fields. These scotomas generally correspond to the sites of arteriolar occlusion or capillary nonperfusion in the retina. The cotton wool spot is the characteristic ophthalmoscopic sign at these areas of ischemia. Angiography with fluorescein clearly demonstrates the areas of capillary nonfilling. In addition to the angiographic evidence, the India ink injection experiments of Ashton indicate rather abrupt interruption of the perfusion of retinal arterioles and their dependent capillary beds. Thus there are a variety of techniques which enable one to conclude that ischemia does play a fundamental role very early in the development of diabetic retinopathy.

One does not need these specialized investigative techniques to convince himself that ischemia underlies the development of diabetic retinopathy. Occluded retinal arterioles, characterized by the silver wire configuration, are often seen, demonstrating by a simple ophthalmoscopic criterion that the early diabetic retina is an ischemic place. In addition, cotton wool exudates are manifestations of ischemic infarcts, and represent, once again, poor vascular perfusion. Thus, we can interpret the diabetic retina as similar to those in the diseases we have previously been considering. This time in the posterior pole, rather than in the peripheral retina, there are focal areas of capillary nonfilling or arteriolar occlusion (Figs. 4-12 and 4-13). With subsequent proliferation, the apparent haphazard arrangement can be deciphered, as Taylor and Dobree [2] have done in London, to indicate that the quadrants of predilection for neovascular responses (to what is presumably the initiating ischemia) are identical to those of sickling's, namely, supratemporal, followed by infratemporal, supranasal, and infranasal. Thus a parallel relationship is again created with the phenomena observed in proliferative sickle retinopathy.

Fluorescein angiography does confirm the marked capillary nonperfusion in

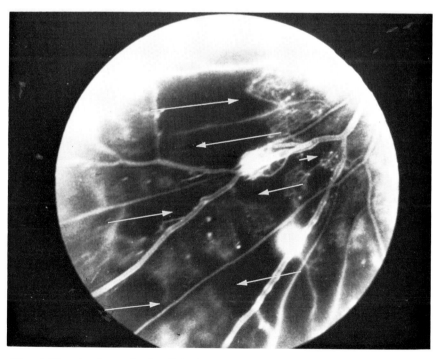

Fig. 4-12. Angiography in diabetic retinopathy. Note widespread areas of focal ischemia (*arrows*) in posterior pole.

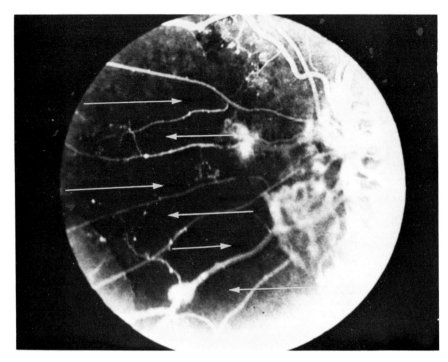

Fig. 4-13. Angiography in diabetes. Note ischemic zones (*arrows*) in posterior pole.

diabetic retinopathy (Figs. 4-12 and 4-13). At the interface of perfused and nonperfused retina one may observe beginning neovascularization. Shunt vessels, or AV anastomoses, probably represent, as in the case of sickling, simple enlargement of preexisting capillaries, because there is no significant transudation or bulk flow of fluorescein from the intravascular space into the vitreous.

One does not *always* observe neovascular tissue flowing into or toward ischemic foci in the diabetic retina; there are sufficient examples of this phenomenon, however (Figs. 4-14 to 4-17), to think that in at least some, if not all, cases the same pathogenetic sequence of events that we have postulated for these other proliferative retinopathies may be applicable to diabetes.

One can speculate that ischemia may be of great significance in many, if not all, of the ophthalmoscopic signs of diabetes. We have already seen, of course, that capillary closure is intimately related to the earliest manifestations of the diabetic process in the retina. In addition, ischemia may be pathogenetically related in a very intimate way to the production of diabetic microaneurysms, since such microaneurysms are often observed immediately adjacent to acellular, nonperfused capillaries. Furthermore, microaneurysms often surround soft exudates or areas of ischemic infarction. The venous dilatation and granular flow that are observed commonly in diabetic retinopathy, it may be conjectured, may be caused, at least in part, by partial obstruction in the distal vascular bed. This, in turn, may represent an ischemic process. Furthermore, hard exudates and retinal edema may represent abnormal permeability of the retinal vessels, which themselves may

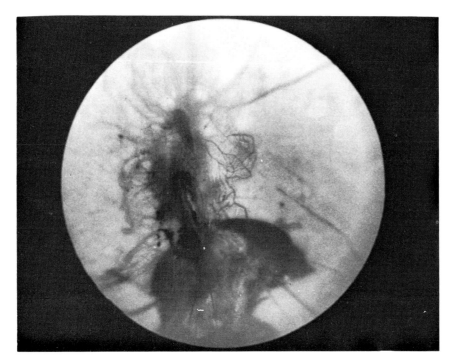

Fig. 4-14. Preangiographic photography of peripapillary neovascularization in diabetes (cf. Fig. 4-15).

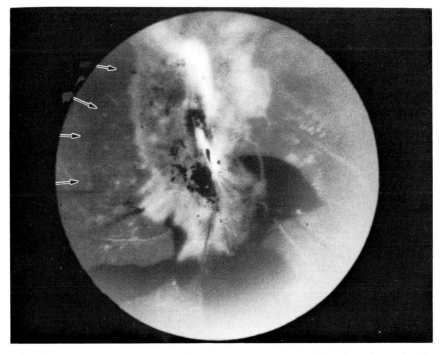

Fig. 4-15. Angiographic view of peripapillary neovascularization shown in Figure 4-14. Note ischemic retina (*arrows*) around neovascular tissue.

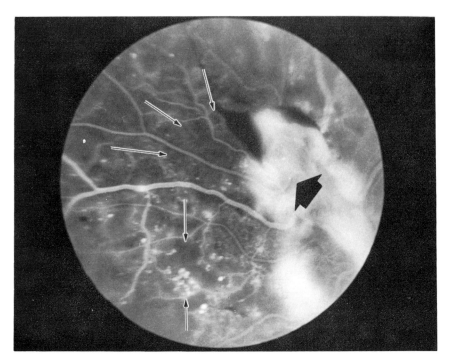

Fig. 4-16. Angiographic view of posterior pole in diabetes. Neovascular tissue (*heavy black arrow*) is growing into an area of ischemic retina (*thin arrows*).

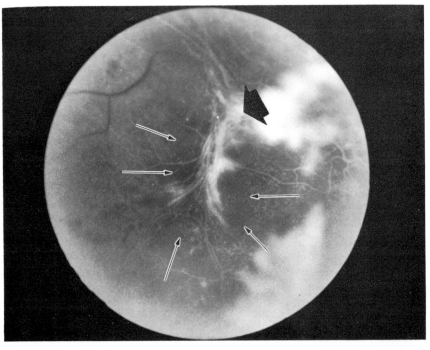

Fig. 4-17. Angiography of the posterior pole in diabetes. Neovascular tissue (*heavy black arrow*) is surrounded by ischemic, nonperfused retina (*thin arrows*).

have become diseased and abnormally leaky by virtue of ischemia-induced damage to their walls.

We have seen in a variety of diseases that neovascularization may represent a reparative effort of new vessels to revascularize ischemic zones. The late regression that is observed in small percentages of all these proliferative diseases may represent a change to even worse ischemia, in which the neovascular tissue itself becomes poorly perfused and therefore becomes infarcted.

Finally, the vitreous contraction that is so significant in the development of vitreous hemorrhage and retinal detachment may also be related to ischemia, since Kloti [3] has indicated in experimental animals that retinal embolization leading to ischemia can itself induce vitreous detachment.

REFERENCES

1. Kohner, EM: The effect of diabetes on retino-vascular function. Acta Diabetologica Latina 8 (Suppl 1):135, 1971
2. Taylor E, Dobree JH: Proliferative diabetic retinopathy. Site and size of initial lesions. Brit J Ophth 54:11, 1970
3. Kloti, R: Experimental occlusion of retinal and ciliary vessels in owl monkeys. I. Technique and clinical observations of selective embolism of the central retinal artery system. Exp. Eye Res 6:393, 1967

Francis I. Caird

Chapter 5
Metabolic Control

If there was ever a contentious subject in general medicine, it is the relationship between the control of diabetes and its complications. For many years it has been an article of faith—and one can use no other word—among some physicians that good control of diabetes can do something to prevent the subsequent development of crippling complications, and many other physicians have equally adopted an attitude of disbelief. Both these attitudes have been put over with the fervor of the proselytizer, and some extremely rigid positions have been taken up. Part of the problem results undoubtedly from the great difficulty that everybody has had in defining what is meant by control of diabetes. There is some difficulty in defining what is meant by the complications of diabetes. The ease of observation of the retina makes it suitable for use as a marker for the microvascular complications of diabetes, and the retina has commonly been so used. There is even difficulty in the definition of diabetes itself. So it is perhaps not surprising that there is still great controversy on this very important matter.

It is now difficult to ignore the evidence that good control of diabetes does, in fact, prevent some of its complications. There are now five adequate studies [2, 5, 8, 12, 13] in which the complications of diabetes are well defined, and so is control of diabetes. All show that control is beneficial. Figure 5-1 illustrates one of these studies.[4] Here the measure of control used is a number called "glycosuria percentage." This is the proportion, expressed as a percentage, of the occasions when on routine clinic attendance the patient's urine sugar was 2 percent or greater; it can be shown that this number is related to the mean blood sugar observed on those same clinic attendance days.[3] This number can serve as a simple and totally unambiguous measure of control for groups of patients, though not for individuals. This is more than can be said for many of the methods of assessing control of diabetes described in the literature. For the study shown in Figure 5-1, 299 patients were selected by the following criteria: all had diabetes, all had the diagnosis of diabetes established in one clinic, all had had an ophthalmic observation 10 to 15 years after the diagnosis of diabetes had been established (the mean duration of diabetes being 12 years), and all had been under the care of one clinic for the entire 10 to 15 years. These patients were then divided into eight groups according to their glycosuria percentage for all 12 years. The

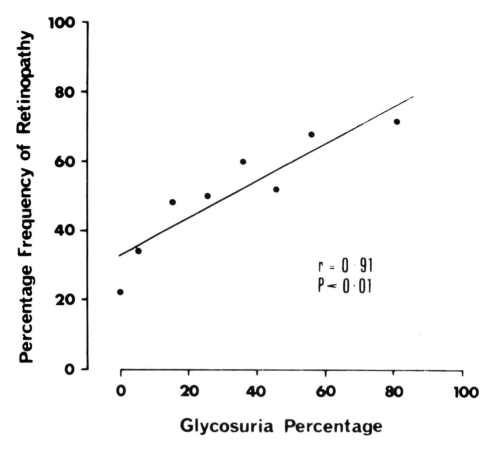

Fig. 5-1. Frequency of retinopathy after 10 to 15 years of diabetes and glyco-suria percentage (Reprinted with permission from Caird FI, Pirie A, Ramsell TG: Diabetes and the Eye. Oxford, Blackwell, 1969).

frequency of retinopathy in each group was determined from the ophthalmic obser-vations, which were made by ophthalmologists, not by general physicians. In the group with the lowest glycosuria percentage, the frequency of retinopathy was just over 20 percent, and in the group with the highest glycosuria percentage, it was over 70 percent. Incidentally, none of these groups is smaller than 20, and the largest of them contains 80 patients. The former group would have had a mean blood sugar at clinic attendance of around 160 mg/100 ml, and the latter of around 320 mg/100 ml. Most physicians would agree that the latter group was badly controlled and the former well controlled, and would view those in between with intermediate degrees of enthusiasm. There is a straight-line relationship between frequency of retinopathy and glycosuria percentage. This is the best evidence to date of a relationship between blood sugar over long periods of time and the sub-sequent frequency of retinopathy.

An interesting observation made by Constam [6] suggested that it may be the first few years after the diagnosis of diabetes that are more critical with respect to the subsequent development of complications, than are the later years. In conse-quence, the 299 patients were redivided according to their glycosuria percentage in the first 5 years after diagnosis, and in the subsequent 7 years. The first 5 years are called the first period and the next 7 years, from the 5th to the 12th year on average, are called the second period. There is a highly significant relationship between the glycosuria percentage in the first period, but no significant relationship between glycosuria percentage between the 5th and 12th years, and the frequency of retinopathy after 12 years (Fig. 5-2). If this conclusion is substantiated by others' work, a number of important things follow. The first is that it provides support for screening programs for diabetes because, clearly, only by early diagnosis can one affect those vital early years. Secondly, it provides support for those who take the view that just because it takes 15 years to develop retinopathy in juvenile diabetes, the diabetes cannot be neglected for 15 years. The third, and perhaps the most important, conclusion is that many of the negative studies are invalidated, in particular the excellent prospective study of Knowles et al.[9] There was no relationship between blood sugar levels and the subsequent development of retinopathy; but a large number of the patients had entered the study more than 5 years after diagnosis, and were therefore quite likely to have been beyond the time when such a relationship could be demonstrated.

The second problem of the relation of metabolic control to retinopathy is the question of whether, once retinopathy is clinically apparent, control of diabetes has any effect. Those who believe that control of diabetes prevents retinopathy sometimes go on to infer that once retinopathy has been established, it is still worth attempting to control diabetes closely in order to prevent progression. This is a logical jump which is not justified, because one could quite easily imagine that local processes in the retina, not under metabolic control in any but the very broadest sense, might take over once retinopathy is apparent, and have an independent life of their own. There is, however, some evidence that even at this stage good control can be beneficial. In the same study [9] it was possible to compare the frequency of malignant retinopathy in relation to glycosuria percentage over the 12-year period, the patients being divided for this purpose into those with high glycosuria percentages (and presumably very high blood sugars for long periods of time) and those with a low glycosuria percentage (Fig. 5-3). The difference is highly significant statistically, despite the fact that it is based on a relatively small number of patients with malignant retinopathy. The same is shown with retinopathy as a whole that the first period seems to be the critical time; the second period apparently does not contribute very much. It would seem to follow that if severe and advanced retinopathy is related to control of diabetes, possibly the progress from slight to severe retinopathy may also be metabolically controlled to some extent. There are several direct studies in the literature.[1, 2, 7, 10, 11] Three of the studies concluded that diabetes is unrelated to progression of retinopathy,[1, 2, 7] two that it is.[10, 11] Perhaps the most convincing study is that of Kohner et al.;[10] about 200 patients were divided into four groups, and the individual major lesions of diabetic retinopathy were considered independently, using photographs and an elegant statistical technique for determining rates of change (Table 5-1). With regard to microaneurysms and hemorrhages, although in all patients taken together there was a highly significant deterioration in the 2-year period over which the study continued, this was not the case in those with very good control. New vessels showed a general tendency to progress, but there was no significant deterioration in any single category of control. Fibrous proliferation, as one might expect,

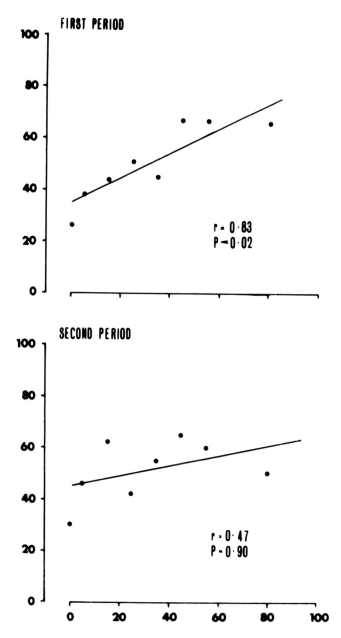

Fig. 5-2. Frequency of retinopathy after 10 to 15 years of diabetes and glycosuria percentage in first period (0 to 5 years approx) and second period (6 to 12 years approx) (Reprinted with permission from Caird FI, Pirie A, Ramsell TG: Diabetes and the Eye. Oxford, Blackwell, 1969).

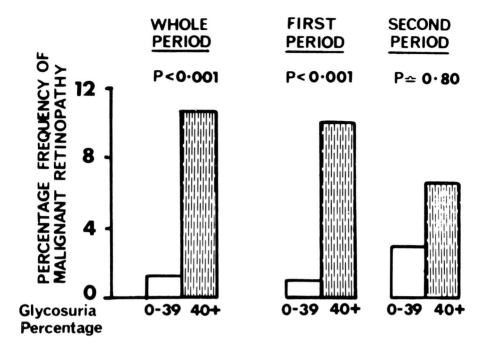

Fig. 5-3. Frequency of malignant retinopathy after 10 to 15 years of diabetes, and glycosuria percentage (Reprinted with permission from Caird FI: In: Goldberg MF, Fine SL (eds): Symposium on the Treatment of Diabetic Retinopathy. US Public Health Service Publ 1890, Washington, 1969).

Table 5-1
Control of Diabetes and Progression of Retinopathy Over 2 years *

Control	Microaneurysms and Hemorrhages	Exudates	New Vessels	Fibrous Proliferation
Very good	−	+ +	−	⎫
Good	+ +	−	−	⎬ + +
Fair	+	−	−	⎰
Poor	+ +	−	−	⎱ +
All	+ +	−	+	+ +

* From Kohner EM, Fraser TR, Joplin GF, Oakley NW: The effect of diabetes control on diabetic retinopathy, in Goldberg MF, Fine, SL (eds): Symposium on the Treatment of Diabetic Retinopathy. US Public Health Service Publ 1890, Washington, 1969.
No significant change   :   −
Deterioration significant at 5-percent level   :   +
Deterioration significant at 1-percent level   :   + +

was unrelated to the degree of metabolic control. There is thus some evidence that some of the lesions of diabetic retinopathy are still, so to speak, under metabolic influence.

Finally, there is a time when severe visual symptoms are present, and the patient is blind or nearly so. There is then often a tendency for physicians to say, "Now, you really must do something about your diabetes and must get it right." Very rigorous dietary restrictions, often taking into account unsaturated fats, etc., may be imposed, and additional forms of metabolic control, such as clofibrate, may be begun. There seems no justification whatever for this at this stage. There is no evidence that anything other than the prevention of purely diabetic symptoms is worthwhile.

In conclusion, I have tried to show that there is factual support for the long-held view that control of diabetes is worthwhile. If two-thirds of diabetic retinopathy is preventable, then diabetic retinopathy is one of the major preventable causes of blindness.

REFERENCES

1. Adnitt PI, Taylor E: Progression of diabetic retinopathy. Relationship to blood sugar. Lancet 1:652, 1970

2. Burditt AF, Caird FI, Draper GJ: The natural history of diabetic retinopathy. Q J Med 37:303, 1968

3. Caird FI: Estimation of the long-term control of diabetes. Diabetes 16:502, 1967

4. Caird FI: In: Goldberg MF, Fine SL (eds): Symposium on the Treatment of Diabetic Retinopathy. US Public Health Service Publ 1890, Washington, 1969, p 142

5. Caird FI, Pirie A, Ramsell TG: Diabetes and the Eye. Oxford, Blackwell, 1969

6. Constam GR: Zur Spätprognose des Diabetes mellitus. Helv Med Acta 32: 287, 1965

7. Gerritzen FM: A Longitudinal Study of Diabetic Retinopathy. Leiden, Nederlandsch Drukkesij Bedrijf, 1970

8. Keiding NR, Root HF, Marble A: Importance of control of diabetes in prevention of vascular complications. JAMA 150:964, 1952

9. Knowles, HC, Guest GM, Lampe J, Kessler M, Skillman TG: The course of juvenile diabetes treated with unmeasured diet. Diabetes 14:239, 1965

10. Kohner, EM, Fraser TR, Joplin GF, Oakley NW: The effect of diabetes control on diabetic retinopathy, in Goldberg MF, Fine SL (eds): Symposium on the Treatment of Diabetic Retinopathy. US Public Health Service Publ 1890, Washington, 1969, p 119

11. Miki E, Fukuda M, Kuzuya T, Kosaka K, Nakao K: Relation of the course of retinopathy to control of diabetes, age, and therapeutic agents in diabetic Japanese patients. Diabetes 18:773, 1969

12. Mohnike G: Zur diabetischen Blutgefasskrankheit. Dtsch Med Wochenschr 82: 1904, 1957

13. Szabo AJ, Stewart AG, Joron GE: Factors associated with increased prevalence of diabetic retinopathy: A clinical survey. Can Med Assoc J 97:286, 1967

Eva M. Kohner

Chapter 6
Retinal Blood Flow in Diabetes Mellitus

Previous papers in this conference (Chapters 2 and 4) have indicated that vascular occlusion resulting in reduced blood flow is responsible for the progression of non-proliferative to proliferative lesions in diabetic retinopathy. These observations are based on clinical appearances and not on measurement of retinal blood flow.

To determine how retinal circulation is altered in diabetes, we have undertaken a study of segmental retinal blood flow in the superior temporal quadrant in nine normal volunteers and 36 diabetic patients.

METHODS

The method used is a modification of that described by Hickam and Frayser [1] who used fluorescein angiography to estimate total retinal blood flow. This method is based on the fact that it is possible to measure the volume flow in a closed vascular bed, provided the volume of the vascular bed and the transit time of blood from the arterial entry point to the venous exit point is known:

$$\text{Volume flow} = \frac{\text{volume of vascular bed}}{\text{transit time}}$$

In the method used, the mean transit time is measured by photographic means, and the volume of the vascular bed is estimated.

Measurement of mean transit time

Hickam and Frayser [1] have shown that when 4 to 5 ml of 5-percent fluorescein is injected into a peripheral vein, the fluorescence emitted from the retinal vessels is proportional to the concentration of fluorescein in those vessels. It has also been shown that if the correct film is used, and care is taken with its development, the antilog of the image density in the photographic negative is proportional to the intensity of the fluorescence (I_f).

We therefore inject 4 ml of 5-percent fluorescein into a peripheral vein and

This work was supported by the Wellcome Trust and the Scientific Section of the British Diabetic Association.

take pictures before the arrival of the dye (for baseline) and then at approximately 1-second intervals while the fluorescein passes through the retinal circulation. The optical density of vessel images is measured from the negative on the baseline film and on each subsequent frame with a scanning densitometer. The intensity of the fluorescence is calculated and plotted against time on semilogarithmic paper. This time-intensity curve has a straight line downslope until recirculation (Fig. 6-1). The straight line to $I_f \times 10 = 1$ is computed by calculating the regression line by the "least squares method." [2]

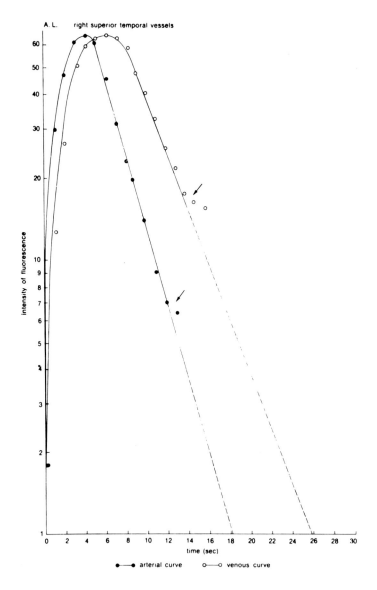

Fig. 6-1. Intensity of fluorescence on logarithmic scale plotted against time for both artery and vein, gives a linear downslope until recirculation of dye (*arrows*) (Reprinted with permission from Kohner EM: Acta Diabetol Lat [Suppl 1] 8:135, 1971).

The mean transit time for both artery and vein is calculated from the areas under the curves obtained:

$$t = \frac{\sum\limits_{n}^{0} I_f(t)t}{\sum\limits_{n}^{0} I_f(t)}$$

where t is the mean circulation time; $I_f(t)$ is the intensity of fluorescence at time t from time 0 to time n; and n is the time at which $I_f = 1$. The mean circulation time t is the difference between tv (mean venous transit time) and ta (mean arterial transit time).

Because the circulation time in different retinal areas is very variable, instead of measuring mean transit time for the whole eye,[1] in this study only the blood flow in the superior temporal quadrant was studied.[2] This measurement is only possible if the assumption is made that the superior temporal vessels form a closed vascular bed, i.e., the supply area of the artery corresponds to the drainage area of the vein.

Estimation of vascular volume

Clearly it is not possible to measure the volume of the vascular bed. Certain assumptions have therefore to be made:

1. Since all the blood reaching the superior temporal segment has to pass through the feeder artery, the cross-sectional area of this artery is related to the blood volume contained in the arterial bed. Similarly, the cross-sectional area of the draining vein reflects the volume of blood in the veins.
2. Since in other organs the approximate distribution of blood volume is 78 percent in the veins, 20 percent in the arteries, and only 2 percent in the capillaries,[1] the volume of the capillary bed can be ignored.

We therefore measured the diameter of the arteries and veins and calculated the cross-sectional area (assuming that this is a circle) on the fluorescein angiograms from those frames which show maximal filling of the retinal vessels. This is probably justified, since in normals there is a linear relationship between mean transit time and cross-sectional area of the vessels ($r=0.746$, $p<0.01$).

Subjects

Nine normal volunteers and 36 diabetic patients were studied on one or more occasions. The diabetic patients were subdivided into three groups: those with mild or no retinopathy (14 patients), those with moderate retinopathy (11 patients, including maculopathy and/or early neovascularisation), and those with severe proliferative lesions (12 patients).

In the normals, one eye only was studied, while in six diabetics mean transit time was measured in both eyes. If the two eyes had retinopathy of the same severity, the mean of the two eyes was taken both for transit time and for volume flow. In 1 patient in whom the two eyes were of different severity, they were considered in their respective group. The two eyes were also considered separately when change in volume flow without or after treatment was studied.

RESULTS

Figure 6-2 shows the volume flow in arbitrary units in the superior temporal quadrant in the normals and three groups of diabetics. Although there was quite a big variation in the normals (range 5.37 to 10.81×10^3 arbitrary units), they were all closely bunched. The variation was much greater in the diabetics, especially in those with mild or no retinopathy (range 8.24 to 37.52×10^3 arbitrary units) and those with moderate lesions (range 2.19 to 36.24×10^3 arbitrary units). In those with severe lesions, the variation was less (range 4.58 to 16.77×10^3

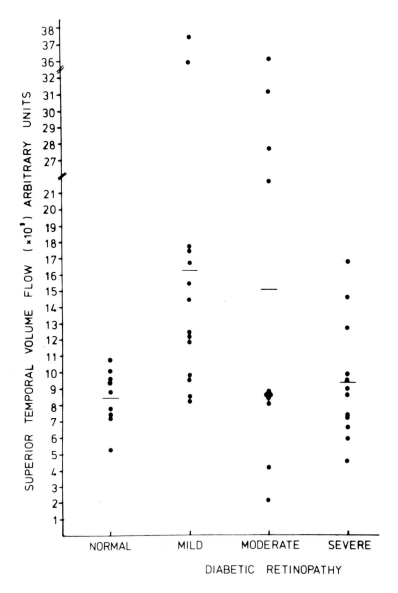

Fig. 6-2. Superior temporal volume flow in arbitrary units in 9 normal subjects and 36 diabetic patients. *Horizontal lines* indicate mean value. Note that the vertical scale is interrupted in two points.

arbitrary units). The mean flow was significantly higher in those with mild or no retinopathy than in normals ($p<0.02$). In those with moderate retinopathy the mean blood flow was twice as high as in normals, but the levels did not reach statistical significance because of the high standard deviation. Only those with the most severe lesions had values similar to the normals (mean 9.45).

Volume flow can only be increased if the vascular volume is increased or the transit time shortened. Contrary to expectation, in this group of patients there was no significant difference in the arterial and venous diameters between normals and diabetics, though for all degrees of retinopathy, diabetic patients had slightly wider vessels.

Considering mean transit time (Fig. 6-3) the situation was different. The mean transit time in patients with no or only early retinopathy was significantly less than in normals ($p<0.01$), though it was similar to that in normals in the other two groups.

There were two further points of interest to us, namely, how repeatable the studies are and what the effect of any specific treatment on volume flow is.

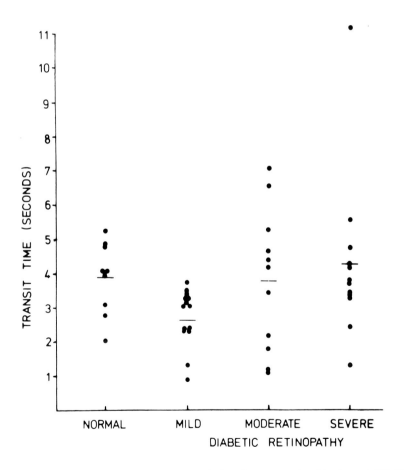

Fig. 6-3. Mean transit time in seconds in nine normal subjects and 36 diabetic patients. *Horizontal lines* indicate mean value.

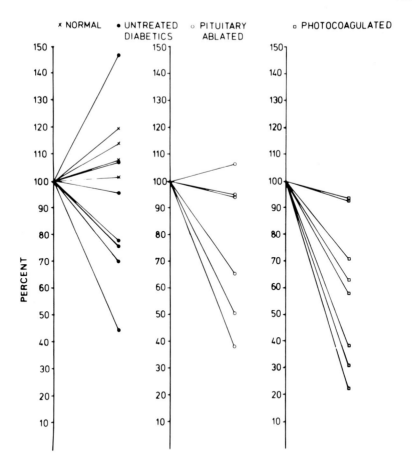

Fig. 6-4. Percent change in change in volume flow between initial and later studies in 4 normals, 7 untreated diabetics (untreated by special means), 6 pituitary-ablated, and 8 photocoagulated patients. Initial study designated as 100 percent.

Figures 6-4 and 6-5 illustrate the change in transit time and volume flow in the groups studied. It shows that in the normals the maximum variation in volume flow was 20 percent between two studies (Fig. 6-4), and 25 percent or less for transit time (Fig. 6-5). In diabetics who were untreated except for their normal diabetic control, the changes were much greater, but because of the great variability and the small number of normals, the results were not significant. Following photocoagulation—a treatment which destroys large retinal areas—the volume flow was decreased in all 7 patients studied. The results almost reach significant levels ($p=0.06$). However, there was no correlation between the reduction of volume flow and the number of photocoagulation applications. Pituitary ablation too, caused a reduction in volume flow in all but 1 patient. The change was less than that seen after photocoagulation. The direction of the change in transit time was in most instances opposite to the changes in volume flow, but there was no good correlation between the two.

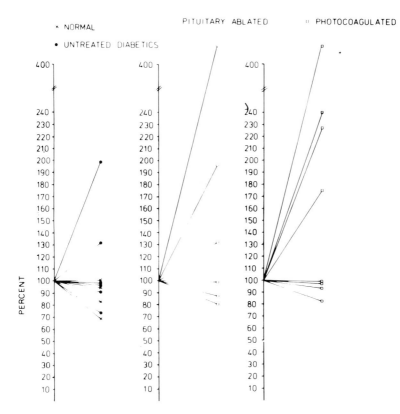

Fig. 6-5. Percent change in transit time between initial and later studies in 4 normals, 7 untreated diabetics, 6 pituitary ablated, and 8 photocoagulated patients. Initial study designated as 100 percent.

DISCUSSION

The results suggest that the volume flow in diabetics is not less but similar to or greater than that seen in normals.

There are several possibilities why the volume flow should be increased in diabetics. The first of these is the presence of shunt vessels, i.e., low-pressure high-flow channels which divert blood from arteries to veins. This is not a very likely reason since shunt vessels have not been demonstrated in those without retinopathy or those with only very mild retinopathy, and it was this group of patients who had the greatest increase in volume flow.

The next possibility is the presence of new vessels. If there are many such vessels with large flow through them, then of course volume flow would be increased. However, this cause can be discarded because those with the most severe lesions did not have an increased volume flow. Also, because of the leakage from the new vessels, those with the most severe lesions in the periphery had to be excluded from the study.

A circulating vasodilator has not been excluded by our work, though the main vessel diameters were similar in normals and diabetics. However, a vasodilator would be more likely to act on terminal arterioles whose diameter cannot be measured accurately.

The most likely cause for the increased blood flow is autoregulation. The term autoregulation is used here in its widest sense, meaning that an organ will adjust its blood flow according to its needs. Diabetes is a metabolic disorder, and it is reasonable to assume that there is accumulation of a normal or abnormal metabolic breakdown product. It is also possible that there is a lack of something —as yet not identified—needed by the retina for normal metabolism. It is this type of "ischemia," rather than that produced by vascular occlusion, which causes increased blood flow in an attempt to supply the missing need.

In the most severe forms of retinopathy, the volume flow would not be increased because the vessels by this time are so diseased that they cannot respond to an autoregulatory demand.

SUMMARY

The retinal blood flow was measured by an indirect method modified from that described by Hickam and Frayser [1] in nine normal volunteers and 36 diabetic patients.

The volume flow was higher in the diabetics as a group than in the normals. The difference only reached statistical significance when those with mild or no retinopathy were compared with normals. These patients also had a significantly lower mean transit time than the healthy controls.

Both pituitary ablation and photocoagulation tended to reduce the volume flow, the change being greater in the photocoagulated eyes.

Autoregulation trying to compensate for the metabolic abnormality of diabetes, is the most likely cause for the increased volume flow.

ACKNOWLEDGMENTS

I would like to thank Professor Russell Fraser for allowing me to study the patients under his care, and Mr. S. J. Saunders and Miss Barbara Sutcliffe for their technical assistance.

QUESTIONS AND ANSWERS

Question. What do you do if you miss the first appearance of fluorescein in these photographs, or for that matter, how do you determine when to stop in order to avoid recirculation?

Dr. Kohner. The first appearance of fluorescein is not a problem. The rise in density is very steep always and, provided I have one or two points before the maximum height of the curve is reached, this is quite adequate for plotting the graph.

As for the recirculation, this, too, is not usually a problem, since the computer plots out the graph and I can therefore see where recirculation occurs and can then direct the computer to integrate, leaving out those points which indicate the recirculation.

Question. Why do you say that the people with high blood sugars have worse controlled diabetes; why don't you say that they just have different diabetes, one of the things about which is that it is more difficult to control?

Dr. Caird. The best I can do is to say that most physicians would agree that by scrupulous attention to detail, virtually every diabetic can be gotten into what would be regarded as a well-controlled state, at least for reasonable periods of time. Certainly one can manipulate my data to show that there are some patients who are well controlled in the first period and badly controlled in the second period; and then there is a group with the sequence reversed. Now they presumably had the same sort of diabetes all the time, but they are at one time more easy to control, at another time less easy to control. They seem to be like leopards changing their spots. That people can change from one category to another is, I think, common experience, and is directly contrary to any hypothesis which suggests that there is a particular separate kind of diabetes, which is very difficult to control.

REFERENCES

1. Hickman JB, Frayser R: Invest Ophthalmol 4:876, 1965
2. Bulpitt CJ, Dollery CT: Cardiovasc Res 5:406, 1971
3. Kohner EM: Acta Diabetol Lat [Suppl. 1] 8:135, 1971
4. Litton A: The Ocular Circulation in Health and Disease. Cant JS (ed). H. Kimpron, 1969, p 18

William L. Hutton

Chapter 7
Retinal Microangiopathy Without Associated Glucose Intolerance

Case reports of diabetic retinopathy without an overt abnormality in carbohydrate metabolism are of interest, both because of their apparent rarity and also because of the implications raised as to the relationship of the angiopathy to metabolic control. In this brief discussion I will present a group of these patients, all of whom demonstrate a retinal picture similar to that seen in diabetes, but without chemical evidence of that disease.

The patients were evaluated medically to rule out the many causes of microaneurysms, as well as underlying problems such as hypertension and renal disease. Ophthalmoscopic consideration was given to these many causes of microaneurysms, such as retinal telangiectasia, vein occlusion, Eales' disease, hemoglobinopathies, and low flow states. Every patient had at least one, and often several, oral plasma glucose tolerance tests. Most of our patients turned out to be quite healthy individuals with no obvious cause for their retinopathy. In order to define more clearly the underlying process, the quadracepts muscle was then biopsied. Using the laboratory and techniques of Dr. Siperstein,[1, 2] the muscle capillary basement membrane (MCBM) thickness was measured. Dr. Siperstein elaborates on his techniques and the basis for this test in Chapter 20. It will suffice to say that most of the major investigators in the problem of basement membrane thickening in diabetes agree that the characteristic sign of diabetic microangiopathy is hypertrophy of the capillary basement membrane. In fact, Williamson states that a presumably normal patient with hypertrophy or abnormal capillary basement membrane must be considered as having the predisposition to diabetes (Table 7-1).[3]

Table 7-1

Width of MCBM	Normals	Diabetics
< 1325 Å	92%	2%
> 1325 Å	8%	98%
> 1600 Å	2%	92%

Table 7-2

Case	Sex	Age	GTT (plasma) F	1	2	Eye	Family History	Muscle Biopsy
(1)	M	38	77	102	84	Microan. in macula	—	1532 ± 106
(2)	F	43	69	110	83	Retinitis proliferans and vitreous hemorrhage	—	2065 ± 167
(3)	M	36	70	152	109	Numerous microan.	—	1932 ± 288
(4)	M	32	89	99	79	Numerous microan.	—	805 ± 57
(5)	M	37	100	145	130	Microan. in macula	Father	1511 ± 138
(6)	M	44	84	190	110	Single microan.	—	2295 ± 166
(7)	F	61	39	126	193	Scattered microan.	Brother and Daughter	1669 ± 119
(8)	F	57	88	158	106	Microan.	Mother, Maternal Grandmother, Maternal Aunt	3739 ± 512

In this study we divided our patients into three groups, utilizing the basement membrane thickness, based on prior work by Dr. Siperstein.[1, 2] We considered an average width of greater than 1325 Å as being suggestive but not diagnostic of diabetes. This is because about 8 percent of normals will fall into this range, while 98 percent of diabetics have this range of basement membrane thickening. We said that anyone with less than 1325 Å width was normal. Any membrane thicker than 1600 Å (which is two standard deviations above the normal mean) we considered as being essentially diagnostic of diabetes, in that only 2 percent of normals would fall into this area, whereas 92 percent of diabetics demonstrate this degree of hypertrophy. Using these criteria, we were able to say that 5 of our 8 patients were in the group considered essentially diagnostic of diabetes, 2 had a basement membrane which we considered suggestive of diabetes, and 1 had a perfectly normal basement membrane. Table 7-2 summarizes our 8 patients. Their retinopathy ranges from a single microaneurysm up to retinitis proliferans. The family history was often positive for diabetes. There is no obvious correlation between the thickness of the basement membrane and the extent of the retinopathy.

CASE HISTORIES

I would like to present three of these cases to illustrate some of the points and give you an example of their fundus appearance.

Case 1. A 38-year-old man complained of blurring of vision in the right eye present for 3 to 4 months prior to seeing us. He had no complaints referable to the left eye. He had a complete medical evaluation which included carotid arteriograms; all tests were normal. There was no family history of diabetes. His pertinent findings were confined to the retina of the right eye. He had hard exudates, retinal edema, and microaneurysms located temporal to the macula in the right eye (Fig. 7-1). The fluorescein study demonstrated the intraretinal edema, cystoid changes and microaneurysms (Fig. 7-2). The width of the patient's basement membrane was found to be 1352 Å, considered to be suggestive but not diagnostic of diabetes.

Discussion. We had 3 patients with the similar retinal picture: unilateral involvement of the macula with microaneurysms and retinal edema; 2 of the 3 had abnormal basement membranes, indicating that there was an underlying abnormality indicative of the prediabetic state. They were all relatively young males, and all pathology was unilateral. This raises the question of retinal telangiectasia. We could not detect any characteristic capillary abnormalities on their fluorescein studies, nor did they have any peripheral fundus evidence of the disease.

Case 2. A 37-year-old black man had been followed in the clinic for 7 years for microaneurysms of unknown etiology in both fundi. He had no family history of diabetes. He has had multiple glucose tolerance tests over this period of time and all have been normal. Multiple sickle cell preps and hemoglobin electrophoreses have been done, and these all demonstrate type AA hemoglobin. His pertinent findings were confined to the retina. Both eyes were involved. He had many microaneurysms scattered throughout each fundus (Fig. 7-3). Fluorescein study confirmed these lesions (Fig. 7-4). His basement membrane was biopsied and

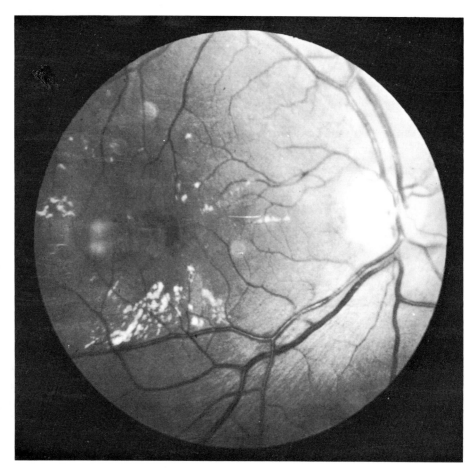

Fig. 7-1.   Case 1. Cluster of microaneurysms, hard exudates. Unilateral findings in man
with normal GTT.

demonstrated a thickened membrane (1932 Å) which is considered essentially
diagnostic of diabetes.

Discussion. An important point this man makes is the extended follow-up. One
frequent and quite valid criticism of cases such as this is that the patients are in
some interlude of normal metabolic homeostasis but in the past they have had a
clearly abnormal carbohydrate tolerance. The 7-year follow-up of this patient,
and what is now a 4-to-5-year follow-up in our other patients, tends to negate
this criticism and indicates our patients are not merely in some interlude of normal
metabolic homeostasis.

Case 3. A 58-year-old woman, had a 3-month history of decreased vision and
metamorphopsia in both eyes. Her medical evaluation was normal. Several
glucose tolerance tests were performed and all were normal. She had a very
strong family history of diabetes; that is, her mother, her grandmother, and a
maternal aunt all had the disease. Her retinopathy consisted of hard exudates,
a few microaneurysms, and some intraretinal vascular abnormalities (Fig. 7-5).
Fluorescein studies illustrate areas of capillary closure, collateral formation,

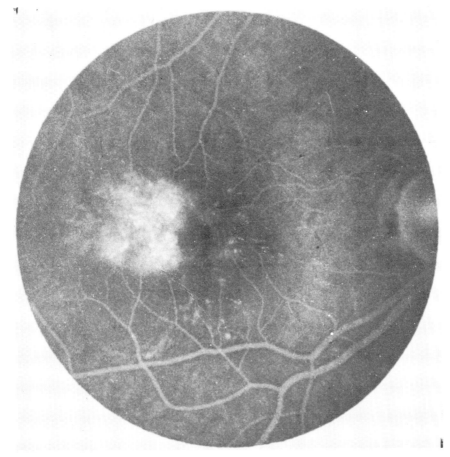

Fig. 7-2. Case 1. Fluorescein study. Many microaneurysms around the macula. Cystoid macular edema.

leakage of dye, and a few microaneurysms (Fig. 7-6). This patient's basement membrane was measured and was found massively thickened (3739Å) which is considered three times that of normal. This membrane is consistent with the diagnosis of genetic diabetes mellitus.

Discussion. There has been a tendency to consider cases of retinal microangiopathy without glucose intolerance as distinctly rare in Diabetes Mellitus. This may be, but these 8 cases, coupled with comments of others in other symposiums, such as Dr. Becker's, would indicate the condition is more common than the scant findings in the literature would seem to reveal.[1] We think these cases are of interest for two reasons: they illustrate that a picture very similar to diabetic retinopathy can occur without the carbohydrate abnormality, and, more importantly, all but 1 patient demonstrated the important associated finding which is characteristic of diabetic microangiopathy—the hypertrophy of their muscle capillary basement membrane.

These cases have raised certain questions about the relationship of retinopathy to metabolic control. Caird has gone into this quite thoroughly in Chapter

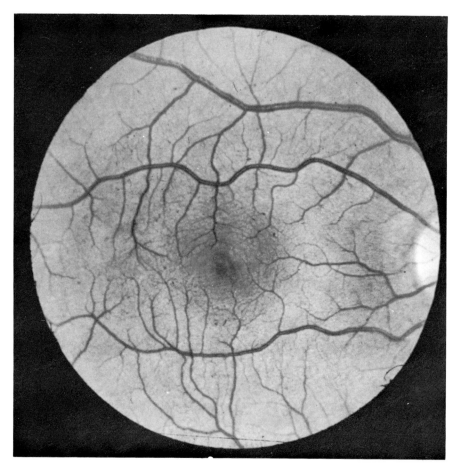

Fig. 7-3. Case 2. Scattered microaneurysms. Other eye had similar lesions.

5.[5] This relationship has been extensively studied, and I think probably any correlation between these aspects of the diabetic syndrome still remains unclear. Dr. Kohner's work certainly indicates that excellent metabolic control, or whatever allows a patient to have excellent metabolic control, will help prevent progression of retinopathy.[6] Dr. Caird and others [7] have indicated that good control early in the development of the carbohydrate problem, before they develop their retinopathy may tend to delay the production of retinopathy. Conversely, other authorities have been unable to demonstrate any significant relationship.[8, 9]

Another method of approaching this problem has been by basement membrane studies, such as Dr. Siperstein's.[1, 2] He has found that 83 percent of prediabetics (defined as someone with a mother and father with unequivocal diabetes, but the patient studied having a normal glucose tolerance) have abnormal MCBM. This would suggest a genetic influence at least on this portion of the microangiopathy. But we can only speculate on the factor or factors regulating the induction of microangiopathy. Certainly, cases such as these suggest that some factor other than metabolic control, at least as we define it now, plays an important role in the formation of retinopathy.

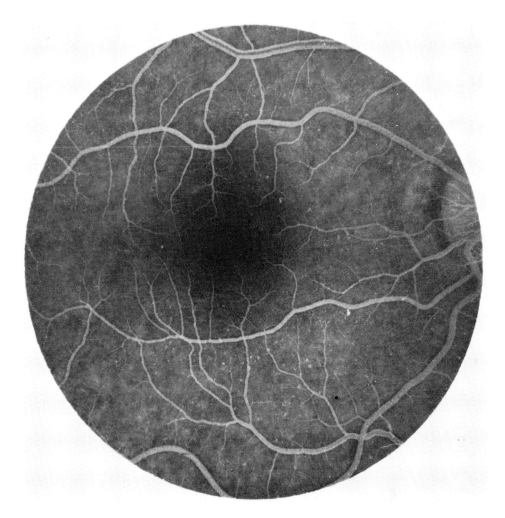

Fig. 7-4.   Case 2. Fluorescein demonstrates microaneurysms.

Besides raising certain theoretical questions concerning the relationship of carbohydrate intolerance to microangiopathy, the measurement of the MCBM emerges as a diagnostic test. As reported by Siperstein,[1,2] and as detailed earlier in this chapter, a thickened capillary basement membrane is very suggestive of genetic diabetes mellitus. This finding is not seen in other causes of increased blood sugar as Cushing's disease, pheochromocytoma, or growth hormone deficient dwarfs,[10] in generalized arteriosclerosis, or in hypertension.[1,2]

There are many causes of ophthalmoscopically visible microaneurysms—such as aortic arch syndrome,[11] or venous-stasis retinopathy,[12] radiation,[13] hemoglobinopathies,[14] and branch vein occlusion—and specific laboratory and clinical tests would allow one to categorize each etiology. Retinal telangiectasis could be a problem, especially if the retinal vessels were rather minimally involved. Certainly the unilaterality which is usually present would be helpful in the diagnosis. Nevertheless, we had 2 patients with a unilateral microangiopathy

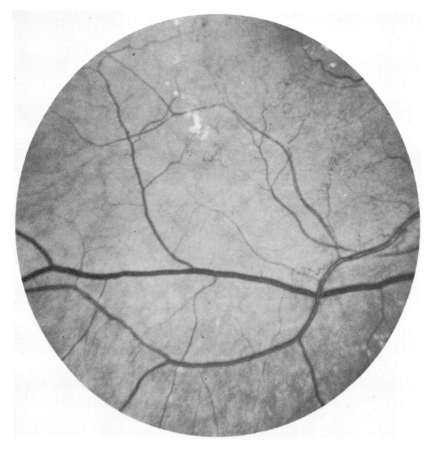

Fig. 7-5. Case 3. Microaneurysms, intraretinal microvascular abnormalities, hard exudates. Other eye has similar lesions.

and abnormally thickened MCBM. The retinal lesions in our cases were micro-aneurysms with localized retinal edema and were not typical of a telangiectasis. Certainly unilateral diabetic retinopathy is unusual, and the association of abnormal MCBM could have been a fortuitous circumstance; yet 2 out of 3 cases are suggestive of a causative relationship.

The typical patient with retinal telangiectasis is a young male with unilateral retinal involvement,[15] although the condition is not uncommonly seen in older persons.[16] One or more foci of dilated, ectatic capillaries are usually found and collateral vessels are often associated with atresia and occlusion of adjacent vessels. The passive congestion and incompetence of these vesseles may lead to exudation and in some cases to progressive detachment of the retina (Coats' disease). Without the fluorescein study, these areas of telangiectasis can mimic microaneurysms. With the fluorescein angiogram one is often surprised to see extensive abnormalities of the capillaries.[17] An occasional patient has more in the way of micro-aneurysmal changes and little or none of the typical telangiectasis. These are the cases in which an evaluation of the MCBM could be of value in establishing the correct diagnosis.

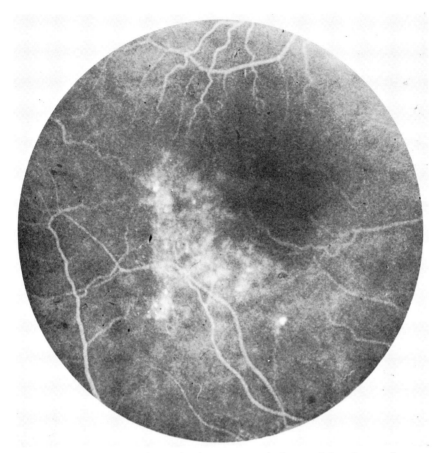

Fig. 7-6.   Case 3. Fluorescein study demonstrates leakage of dye from microvascular abnormalities.

Diabetic retinopathy, with or without overt glucose intolerance, has an important associated finding of hypertrophy of the MCBM, indicating a diabetic or prediabetic state underlying the retinal pathology. The retinopathy, the normal glucose tolerance, and the muscle capillariopathy form a complex which suggests that some factor or factors other than just the metabolic aspects we now recognize must influence the formation of retinopathy.

REFERENCES

1. Siperstein MD, Norton W, Unger RH, Madison LL: Muscle capillary basement membrane width in normal, diabetic, and prediabetic patients. Trans Assoc Am Physicians 79:330, 1966
2. Siperstein MD, Unger RH, Madison LI: Studies of the muscle capillary basement membrane in normal subjects, diabetic, and prediabetic patients. J Clin Invest 47:1973, 1968
3. Williams JR, Volger NJ: Symposium of diabetes mellitus. Med Cl N Am 55: 847, 1971
4. Becker B: In Conference on diabetic retinopathy. Surv Ophthalmol, vol 6: 483, 1961
5. Caird F: Control of diabetes and diabetic retinopathy. In Goldberg FM, Fine SL (eds): Symposium on the Treatment of Diabetic Retinopathy. US Public Health Service Publ 1890, Washington, 1969, p. 107

6. Kohner EM, Fraser TR: The effect of diabetic control on diabetic retinopathy. In Goldberg MF, Fine SL (eds): Symposium on the Treatment of Diabetic Retinopathy. US Public Health Service Publ 1890, Washington, 1969, p. 119

7. Miki E, Fukuda M: Relations of course of retinopathy to the control of diabetic, age, and therapeutic agents in diabetic Japanese patients. Diabetes 18:73, 1969

8. Knowles HC: The control of diabetes mellitus and the progression of retinopathy. In Goldberg MF, Fine SL (eds): Symposium on Treatment of Diabetic Retinopathy. US Public Health Service Publ 1890, Washington, 1969, p. 115

9. Admitt PI, Taylor E: Progression of diabetic retinopathy. Lancet 1:652, 1970

10. Merimee TJ. Siperstein MD, Fineberg SE, McKusick VA: The microangiopathic lesions of diabetic mellitus; an evaluation of possible causative factors. Trans Assoc Am Physicians 132:102, 1970

11. Hedges TR: The aortic arch syndrome. Arch Ophthalmol 71:28, 1964

12. Kearns TP, Hollenhorst RW: Venous-stasis retinopathy in occlusive disease of the carotid artery. Mayo Clin Proc 38: 304, 1963

13. Chee PHY: Radiation retinopathy, Am J Ophthalmol 99:860, 1968

14. Goodman G, Von Sallman L, Holland MG: Ocular manifestation of sickle cell disease. Arch Ophthalmol 58:635, 1957

15. Reese AB: Telangiectasis of the retina and Coats' disease. Am J Ophthalmol 42:1, 1956

16. Henkind P, Morgan G: Peripheral retinal angioma with exudative retinopathy in adults (Coats' lesion). Br J Ophthalmol 50:2, 1966

17. Gass JDM: A Fluorescein angiographic study of macular dysfunction secondary to retinal vascular disease. V. Retinal telangiectasis. Arch Ophthalmol 80:592, 1968

Morton F. Goldberg

Chapter 8

Electron Microscopic Appearance of Argon Laser Burns in the Human Retina and Optic Nerve

Over the past 1.5 years, Dr. David Apple, Dr. George Wyhinny, and I have had the opportunity of experimentally treating several human eyes and several monkey eyes, with argon laser burns of various types in an attempt to determine the histologic and electron microscopic appearances of the argon laser burn in the primate retina. I would like to demonstrate the nature of the variety of burns we have placed. We have attempted to simulate burns that one might create in clinical circumstances. The human eyes that will be presented represent patients with malignant melanoma who consented to undergo photocoagulation with the argon laser prior to enucleation. In all cases, single burns in individual locations were used, and the eyes were enucleated 24 hours after the burns. Burns of different spot size were placed directly over arterioles and venules of different diameters. Multiple burns were placed in the macular region, and you will note something that I believe Dr. Little and Dr. Zweng first pointed out at their initial argon laser course, namely, that when one photocoagulates in the center of the fovea, the intensity of the coagulation is greater than in the perifoveal areas (Fig. 8-1), even though the parameters set on the delivery system of the laser are unchanged.

A variety of "painting" lesions has also been placed. The site in Fig. 8-2 is over the melanoma itself (Fig. 8-2). You will note definite interruption of the blood vessels. As you will see from the electron microscopic material, this has been the only location where we have been able to induce permanent interruption of the normal vascular column under these specified experimental conditions (for details, see Apple DJ., Goldberg MF., and Wyhinny G., Am J Ophth 75:595-609, 1973).

In delivering the burns, the intensity was gradually increased to a point where spasm of a treated vessel was induced; by clinical criteria, it appeared that the vascular column was interrupted. Twenty-four hours later, the vessel characteristically had completely opened up. On fluorescein angiography distal to the burns (Fig. 8-3) one can see normal perfusion and the typical appearance of the vascular burn with marked transudation of the intravascular dye. A similar phenomenon over the acute burn was observed in the vessels of the disc itself (Fig. 8-4).

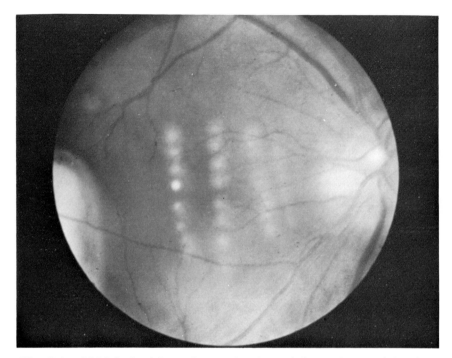

Fig. 8-1. Multiple focal burns in macula. Same delivery characteristics, but note more intense coagulation in center of fovea.

Coagulated tissue was fixed for electron microscopy and imbedded in plastic. In contradistinction to ordinary formalin fixation and hematoxylin-eosin staining, one has an extremely good idea of the number of capillaries in the nerve fiber layer when tissue is prepared in this manner (Fig. 8-5); with routine fixation and staining, capillaries ordinarily are not as easily visible. The status of capillaries and their surrounding nerve fibers may be difficult or impossible to ascertain without electron microscopy. The arterioles and venules also lie within the nerve fiber layer of the retina.

I would now like to make two major points in this presentation. The first is that it is considerably less easy to close normal retinal arterioles and capillaries permanently with the argon laser than one might initially have believed; and the second is that it is considerably easier than expected to induce necrosis in the nerve fiber layer around these vessels (both in the retina and in the optic nerve). If, in fact, the hemoglobin in the capillary bed preferentially absorbs argon wavelengths, one might assume, a priori, that heat could be transmitted to the nerve fiber layer structures.

Electron microscopy of one of the "painted" lesions on the major supratemporal pair of vessels is shown in Figure 8-6. This area of retina shows essentially total cystoid degeneration with marked necrosis involving all layers of the retina. This burn was created with 400 mW, a 100μ spot size, and the duration of exposure was several seconds. The "painting" was continued until visible spasm occurred in the supratemporal vessels. With this intensity burn, there is marked degeneration of full-thickness retina, but the vessel itself remains intact.

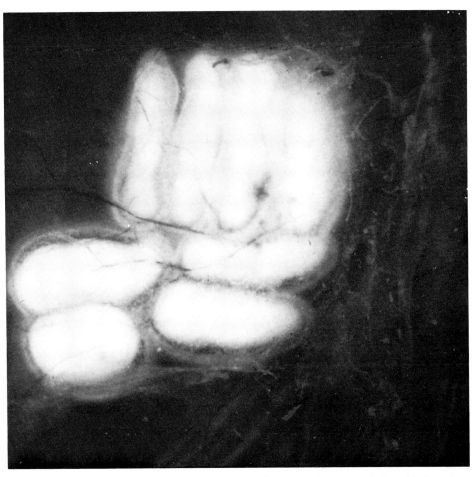

Fig. 8-2. "Painted" argon burns over malignant melanoma of choroid (enucleation specimen). (Reprinted with permission from Apple DJ, Goldberg MF, Wyhinny G,
Levi S: Argon laser photocoagulation of choroidal malignant melanoma. Arch Ophthalmol 90:97–101, 1973).

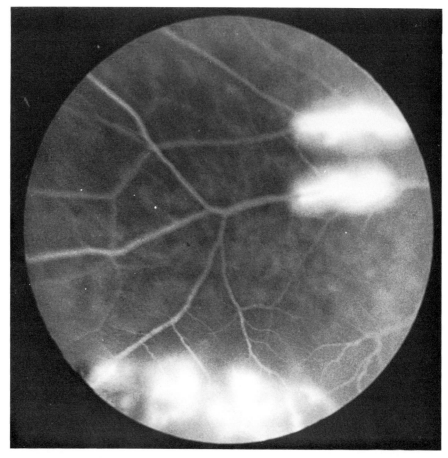

Fig. 8-3. Distal to "painted" burns over superotemporal vessels, fluorescein angiography confirms persistent patency of vessels. Note transudation through vascular walls at burn sites, immediately following photocoagulation. (Reprinted with permission from Apple DJ, Goldberg MF, Wyhinny G: Histopathology and ultrastructure of the argon laser lesion in human retinal and choroidal vasculatures. Am J Ophth, 75: 595–609, 1973).

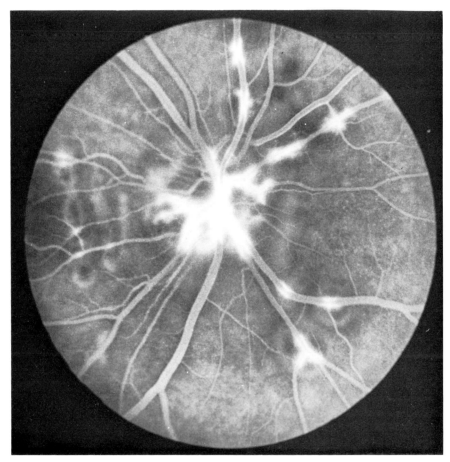

Fig. 8-4. Immediately following argon photocoagulation of disc and peripapillary vessels, marked transudation occurs through walls of burned vessels. (Reprinted with permission from Apple DJ, Goldberg MF, Wyhinny G: Histopathology and ultrastructure of the argon laser lesion in human retinal and choroidal vasculatures. Am J Ophth, 75:595–609, 1973).

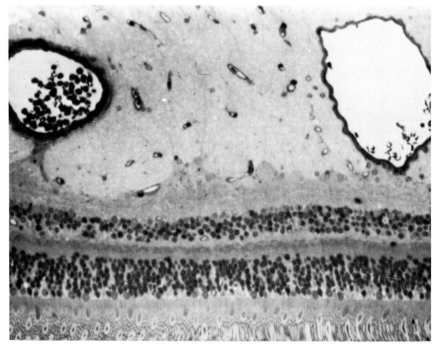

Fig. 8-5. Retina fixed for electron microscopy, embedded in plastic and stained with Mallory blue reveals full extent of innumerable capillaries in nerve fiber layer. (Reprinted with permission from Apple DJ, Goldberg MF, Wyhinny G: Histopathology and ultrastructure of the argon laser lesion in human retinal and choroidal vasculatures. Am J Ophth, 75:595–609, 1973).

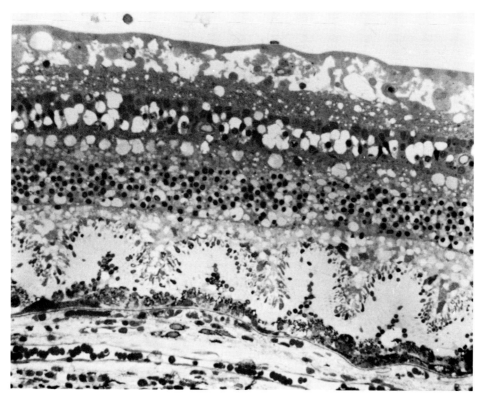

Fig. 8-6. Electron microscopic appearance of "painted" superotemporal vessel. Marked retinal damage has occurred, but the vessel itself, not seen in this section, remains patent (cf. Fig. 8-3).

Figure 8-7 shows a rather typically appearing coneshaped lesion created by a mild to moderate burn. The particular burn that is illustrated was created with 200 mW and a 100-μ beam diameter for 0.2 seconds of exposure. The pyramid or coneshaped configuration is very characteristic; beginning with its apex at the arteriole within the nerve fiber layer, the surrounding damage involves the nerve fiber layer, and there is a spreading out of the damage into the deeper portions of the retina, the pigment epithelium, and even into the choriocapillaris. Although there is periarteriolar degeneration to a rather marked extent, the arteriole itself remains quite patent.

Figure 8-8 shows the retina of a monkey that had a moderate to slightly intense burn; 500 mW were delivered for 0.2 seconds with a 100-μ beam diameter. There is marked necrosis of the periarteriolar retina, but note that the arteriole itself looks remarkably normal. There is minimal cystoid change in its wall, but there is a completely patent lumen.

In Figure 8-9 we see what might be considered a desirable microscopic appearance of blood vessels following argon laser burns. Both in a capillary and in an arteriole, there is marked thrombosis and plugging of the lumen of the vessels with fused erythrocytes. In our experimental human material, this repre-

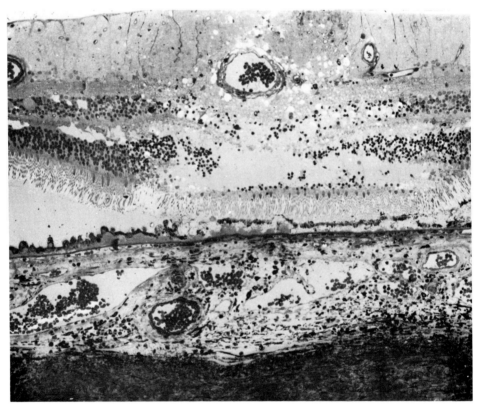

Fig. 8-7. The typical coneshaped full-thickness argon burn in the retina is shown following a mild-moderate burn. (Reprinted with permission from Apple DJ, Goldberg MF, Wyhinny G: Histopathology and ultrastructure of the argon laser lesion in human retinal and choroidal vasculatures. Am J Ophth, 75:595–609, 1973).

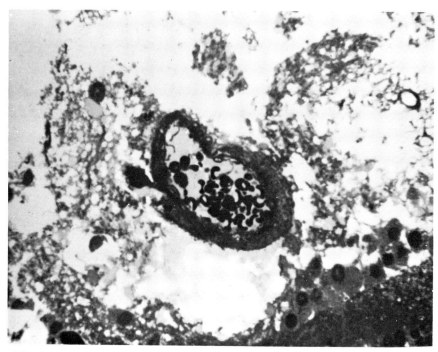

Fig. 8-8. Moderately intense retinal burn. Note periarteriolar necrosis but relatively normal arteriole.

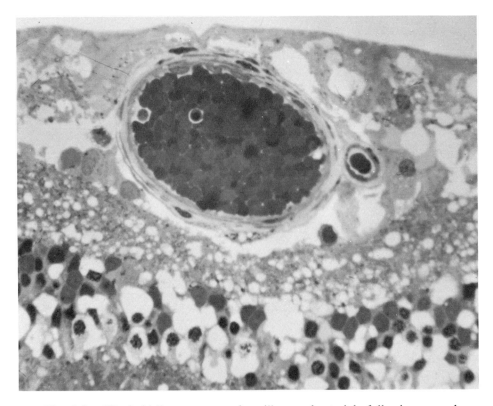

Fig. 8-9. "Desirable" appearance of capillary and arteriole following argon burn, i.e., plugging of vascular lumen with fused erythrocytes. (Reprinted with permission from Apple DJ, Goldberg MF, Wyhinny G, Levi S: Argon laser photocoagulation of choroidal malignant melanoma. Arch Ophthalmol 90:97–101, 1973).

sents one of the few examples we have of such "favorable" results; this particular coagulation was created over the pigmented melanoma, where it might be presumed that additional heat was generated by absorption of light by the pigmented tissue.

The particular lesion in Figure 8-10 was created by a mild burn; I think that therapists would agree that one can define this burn as "mild," i.e., 100 mW for 0.2 seconds with a 50-μ beam diameter. Note the normal arteriole, but the marked cystoid degeneration in the retina. Of even more significance, perhaps, is the fact that a capillary remains totally patent and uninvolved even though it is immediately adjacent to this markedly degenerated retina. Another example of a mild burn is shown in Figure 8-11. This burn was created with 50 mW for 0.2 seconds with a 50-μ beam diameter. Once again the capillary looks essentially normal even though it is surrounded by marked cystoid degeneration and necrosis of the surrounding retina.

Increased burn intensity is shown in Figure 8-12. A moderate burn (300 mW for 0.2 seconds with a 100-μ beam diameter) has slightly damaged a capillary lying adjacent to a coagulated cystoid space. Despite slight damage, the capillary remains open; it was carrying blood at the time of enucleation.

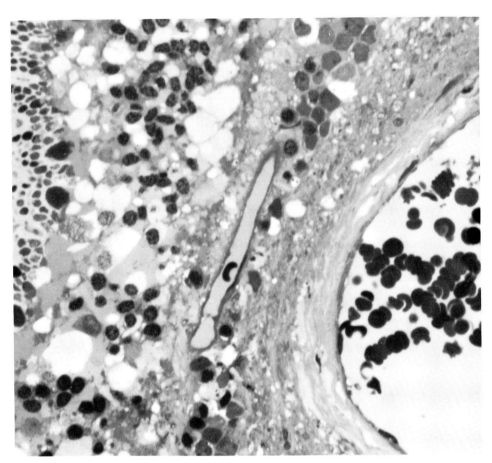

Fig. 8-10. Mild retinal burn. Note patent capillary and arteriole surrounded by marked retinal degeneration. (Reprinted with permission from Apple DJ, Goldberg MF, Wyhinny G: Histopathology and ultrastructure of the argon laser lesion in human retinal and choroidal vasculatures. Am J Ophth, 75:595–609, 1973).

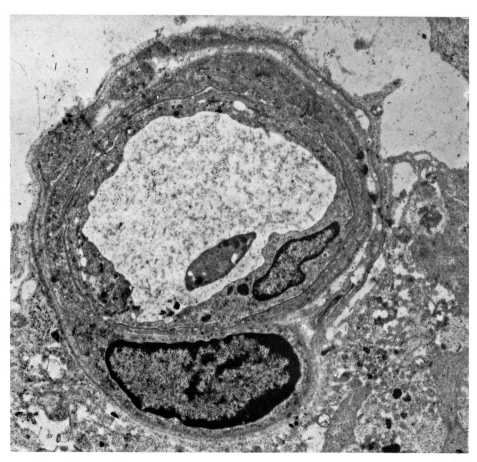

Fig. 8-11. Mild retinal burn. Capillary is essentially normal, despite surrounding necrosis. (Reprinted with permission from Apple DJ, Goldberg MF, Wyhinny G: Histopathology and ultrastructure of the argon laser lesion in human retinal and choroidal vasculatures. Am J Ophth, 75:595–609, 1973).

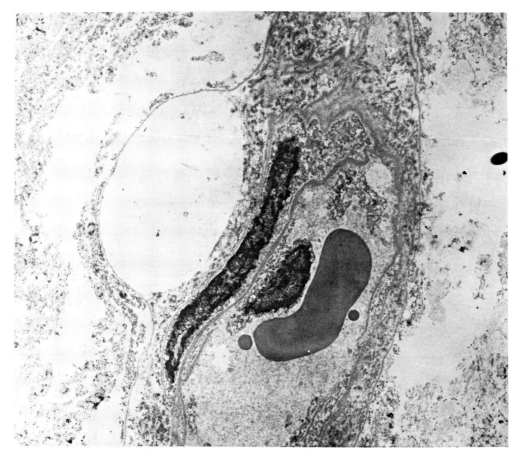

Fig. 8-12. Moderate retinal burn. Note slight damage to capillary wall, but patent capillary lumen and surrounding retinal destruction. (Reprinted with permission from Apple DJ, Goldberg FM, Wyhinny G: Histopathology and ultrastructure of the argon laser lesion in human retinal and choroidal vasculatures. Am J Ophth, 75:595–609, 1973).

The effects of slightly more energy are seen in Figure 8-13, where a 400-mW burn was applied for 0.2 seconds with a 100-μ beam diameter. Now we see what might be presumed to be a hoped-for effect, namely, fused erythrocytes and a totally plugged capillary lumen.

In the case of the optic nerve, it has been considered that this might be one of the safest places to use an argon laser because of its seeming lack of pigmentation. Hence, one might suppose that less light is absorbed, and that consequently less energy is converted to thermal and coagulative effects. In the human optic nerve shown in Figure 8-14, a reasonably mild burn has been placed (100 mW for 0.2 seconds with a 100-μ beam diameter). There is marked necrosis of the nerve fiber layer near the disc. One could explain the necrosis in this particular section by suggesting that heat was transmitted to the nerves from the peripapillary pigment epithelium, but we have recreated this type of lesion by photocoagulating immediately in the center of the optic nerve. It is therefore reasonable to conclude

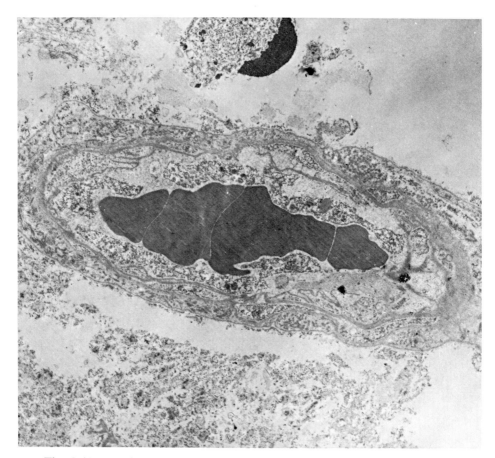

Fig. 8-13. Moderate retinal burn. Note fused erythrocytes and plugged capillary lumen. Reprinted with permission from Apple DJ, Goldberg MF, Wyhinny G: Histopathology and ultrastructure of the argon laser lesion in human retinal and choroidal vasculatures. Am J Ophth, 75:595–609, 1973).

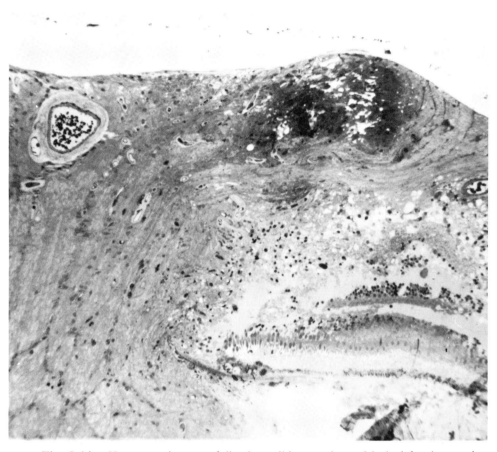

Fig. 8-14.   Human optic nerve following mild argon burn. Marked focal necrosis of nerve fibers has occurred. (Reprinted with permission from Apple DJ, Goldberg MF, Wyhinny G: Histopathology and ultrastructure of the argon laser lesion in human retinal and choroidal vasculatures. Am J Ophth, 75:595–609, 1973).

that it is feasible, with mild argon laser burns, to cause significant necrosis in nonpigmented optic nerve tissue. To show the full extent of this potential, a monkey optic nerve has been heavily photocoagulated (Fig. 8-15). One ordinarily would never employ such an intense burn in clinical circumstances. Total necrosis of the optic nerve in this area has been created by 800 mW for 0.2 seconds with a 100-μ beam diameter. By electron microscopy of the optic nerve, one can see normal configurations in an untreated area (Fig. 8-16) and, by comparison, total destruction in the area of laser photocoagulation (Fig. 8-17).

In summary, therefore, I have tried to make two major points: (1) it is considerably less easy than one might expect to occlude normal vascular tissues in the human and primate retina with argon laser photocoagulation; and (2) it is considerably easier than expected to create damage to the peri-vascular retinal nerve fiber layer and optic nerve.

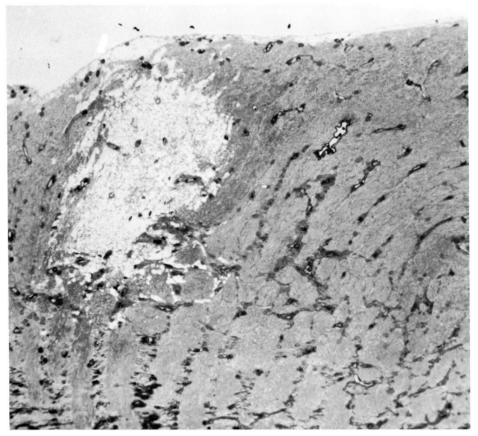

Fig. 8-15.   Monkey optic nerve following intense argon burn. Note massive destruction in nerve.

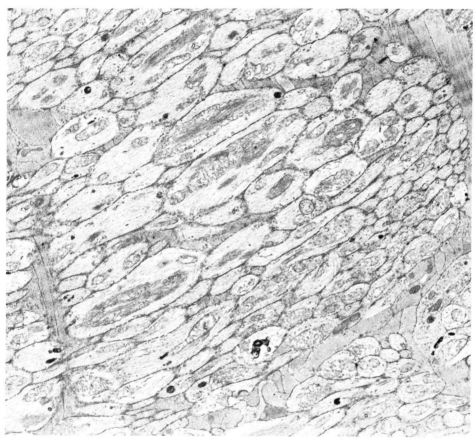

Fig. 8-16.   Normal electron microscopic appearance of monkey optic nerve (cf. Fig. 8-17).

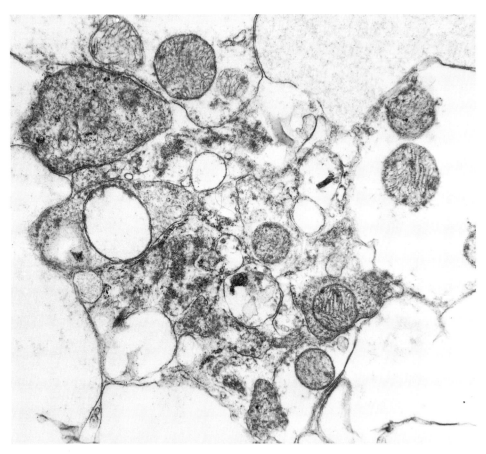

Fig. 8-17.   Intense burn to monkey optic nerve destroys most of nerve fibers (cf. Fig. 8-16).

H. Christian Zweng

Chapter 9

Selection of Cases of Diabetic Retinopathy for Treatment by Argon Laser Slit-Lamp Photocoagulation

In reflecting upon the assignment given to me, I thought that I owed it to the participants not only to indicate the types of cases we are treating, but to indicate how we are treating them. There are three methods of treatment by photocoagulation of diabetic retinopathy: (1) treatment of focal pathology, (2) treatment of the proliferating vessels by coagulation of the feeder vessel(s) and then of the frond, and (3) the treatment of the relatively hypoxic retina by widespread peripheral retinal photocoagulation, hopefully to put blood supply and oxygen demand in better relationship to each other, not only to get rid of the present neovascularization, but to prevent future neovascularization. The treatment of focal pathology is coagulation of "everything that's red": blot or dot hemorrhages, microaneurysms, and the neovascular tufts in the plane of the retina and leaking points as demonstrated by retinal fluorescein angiography. The treatment to the feeder vessel(s) and then to the frond is done by identification of the feeder vessel(s) that serve the neovascular frond by fluorescein angiography. This is especially useful when the neovascularization presents into the vitreous from either the nerve head or from the plane of the retina. Coagulation of the feeding vessel is done until vascular flow is interrupted and then the neovascular frond itself is photocoagulated. The third treatment form (of relative retinal hypoxia) is widespread peripheral retinal photocoagulation. I do not like the word "ablation," because we do not "blot out" the retina, and "barrage" is incorrect. If someone has a shorter way to say "widespread peripheral retinal photocoagulation," I would like to hear it. Photocoagulation is done from the nerve head to the equator except in the macula or maculopapillary bundle. Focal coagulation is also done in the macula and maculopapillar bundle.

The classification of diabetic retinopathy that Dr. Little and I have developed is shown in Table 9-1. It is not a complete classification of diabetic retinopathy. It does not include vitreal hemorrhages, retinal separations, and so on, but for photocoagulation it is a useful and simple classification.

We rarely treat grade 1a, that is, nonproliferative retinopathy without macu-

Table 9-1

Classification of Diabetic Retinopathy for Photocoagulation

Grade	
1	Nonproliferative
	a Background retinopathy without macular edema
	b Background retinopathy with macular edema, localized leakage
	c Background retinopathy with macular edema, diffuse leakage
2	Neovascularization in the plane of the retina
3	Neovascularization into the vitreous or on the nerve head
4	Grade 3 plus glial and/or fibrous tissue proliferation

lar edema. These patients have normal vision; if their vision is impeded, it is not because of retinopathy.

We use focal photocoagulation in grades 1b, 1c, localized leakage (grade 1b) and diffuse leakage, occupying virtually the whole posterior pole (grade 1c). We also treat neovascularization in the plane of the retina and neovascularization into the vitreous or on the nerve head (grades 2 and 3). Neovascularization into the vitreous from the nerve head gives the worst prognosis, and any form of therapy of diabetic retinopathy must markedly reduce or abolish disc neovascularization to be termed "effective." We have used focal coagulation directly upon disc neovascularization; sometimes it rids the nerve head of it and sometimes not. Occasionally hemorrhage occurs and sometimes there is a nerve fiber defect, especially on repeated treatments. So, we are treating grade 3 cases in different ways now. We seldom treat grade 4, cases in which blood supply and oxygen demand have achieved a balance "spontaneously." The nerve head is atrophic, the arteries are narrowed. If there is neovascularization, it is minimal and imbedded in glial and fibrous tissue, usually in the arc along the superior and inferior vascular arcades.

Figure 9-1 is an example of grade 1a with a benign amount of diabetic retinopathy; there are several leaking microaneurysms with a collarette of lipoproteinaceous material and localized intraretinal edema, but since the macula is not involved and the patient is seeing 20/20, no treatment was indicated or given. Even with a good deal more background retinopathy we do not treat these unless central vision is interfered with.

Figure 9-2A shows a case of grade 1b in which there is a good deal of background retinopathy and decrease in central vision, as in this case with 20/80 vision; photocoagulation was done to "everything that is red" and to leaks seen in the fluorescein angiogram. Seven months later visual acuity was 20/25 after three photocoagulation sessions were carried out (Fig. 9-2B). Figure 9-3A shows more lipid deposits from intraretinal leaks and visual acuity of 20/30–. The angiogram (Fig. 9-3B) shows, as is so often the case, the major area of leakage and pathology temporal from the macula. After three sessions of focal photocoagulation, vision improved to 20/20+1 although the patient still shows some lipoproteinaceous material and has a new little hemorrhage temporal from the macula (Fig. 9-3C), illustrating that these patients must be kept under surveillance

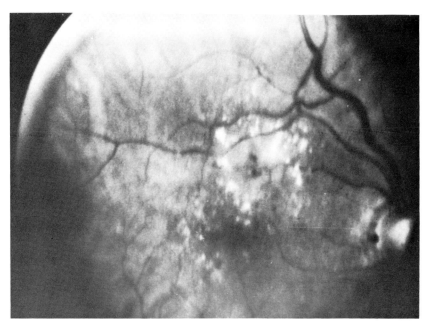

Fig. 9-1.   Grade la diabetic retinopathy showing several leaking microaneurysms with collarette of lipoproteinaceous material and localized intraretinal edema. Visual acuity 20/20.

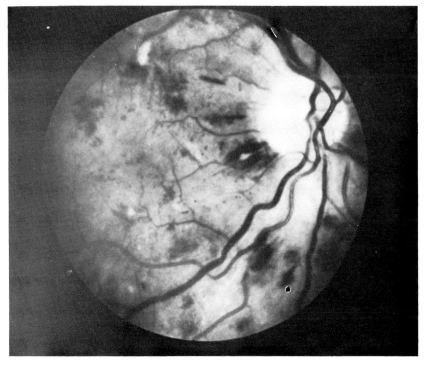

Fig. 9-2A.   Diabetic retinopathy grade 1b showing background retinopathy and localized retinal edema. Visual acuity 20/80 (cf. Fig. 9-2B).

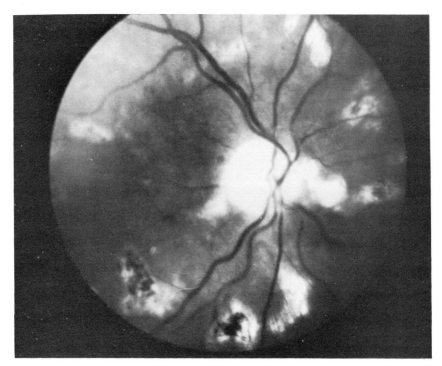

Fig. 9-2B. Same case as Figure 9-2A, 7 months after photocoagulation. There is no intraretinal edema. Visual acuity 20/25.

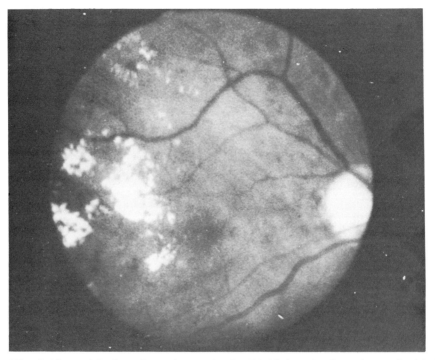

Fig. 9-3A. Diabetic retinopathy grade 1b. Lipid deposits from intraretinal leaks from microaneurysms. Visual acuity 20/30–1 (cf. Figs. 9-3B and 9-3C).

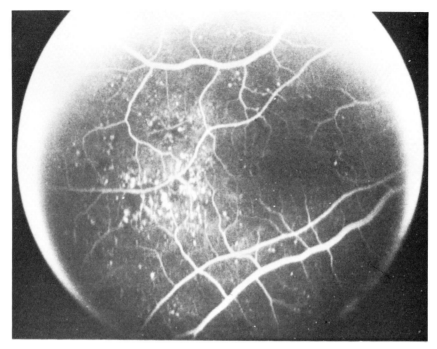

Fig. 9-3B. Fluorescein angiogram of same patient as in Figure 9-3A showing the major area of pathology temporal from the macula (cf. Fig. 9-3C).

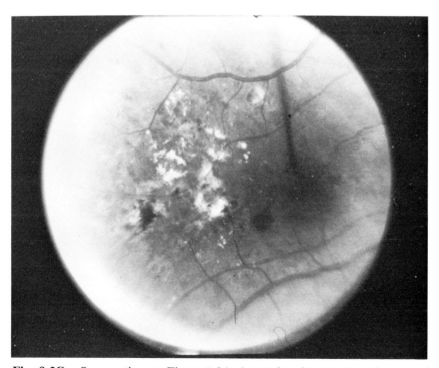

Fig. 9-3C. Same patient as Figure 9-3A, 3 months after treatment began. Visual acuity 20/20+1. Some lipoproteinaceous material is still present and a new small hemorrhage can be seen temporal from the macula.

indefinitely. In Figure 9-4A there is a classical, large, succulent leaking micro-aneurysm in the macula; one does not need a fluorescein angiogram to know that the microaneurysm is leaking: it has a collarette of lipoidal material. Figure 9-4B is immediately postop to show how close to the fovea we photocoagulate, no closer than 200 μ.

An example of grade 1c is seen in Figure 9-5A. There is intraretinal edema involving the whole posterior pole with visual acuity of 20/400. Such eyes have visual acuity of 20/100 to hand motions. When the edema clears with treatment to the focal pathology, the best visual acuity attained is 20/80; 20/200 is not unusual. There is no microcystic macular edema in the same patient (Fig. 9-5B) taken 6 months later. Macular hyperpigmentation at the level of the retinal pigment epithelium (RPE) is almost invariably present; it is a prognostic sign that the best visual acuity to expect is 20/100 to 20/200.

Grade 2 (Fig. 9-6A) shows a neovascular tuft just above the nerve head before treatment with direct argon laser photocoagulation; Figure 9-6B shows the area immediately after treatment with most of the tuft obliterated. Figure 9-6C shows the same area 1 month later; the tuft is gone. Figure 9-7A shows two areas of neovascularization on the retina. In the two areas 2 months after treatment, pigmentation has replaced the tufts (Fig. 9-7B). Such tufts are not hard to obliterate because the structures to be coagulated are close to the RPE which has, of course, many melanin granules to absorb the light and radiate heat. Sometimes such areas must be treated several times: the first time to develop hyperpigmentation in the area and destroy part of the neovascularization and a

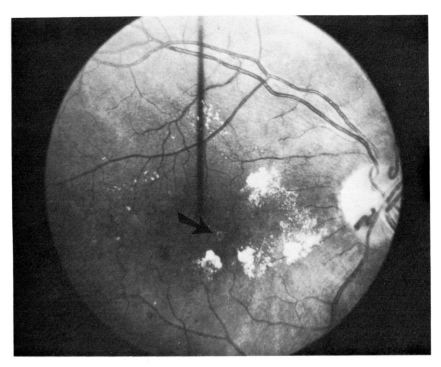

Fig. 9-4A. Diabetic retinopathy grade 1b. Arrow indicates a large leaking microaneurysm with collarette of lipid (cf. Fig. 9-4B).

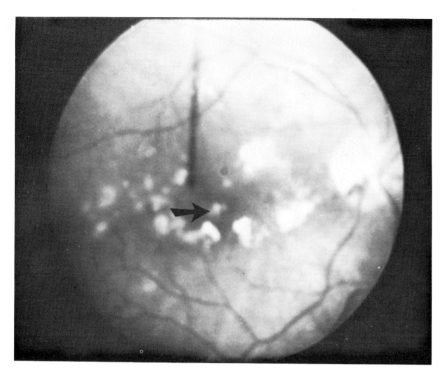

Fig. 9-4B. Same patient as Figure 9-4A immediately after argon laser photocoagulation. The microaneurysm has been photocoagulated with 50-μ spot size, 0.1 second time exposure, 150 mW power. Treatment should be given no closer to the fovea than 200 μ.

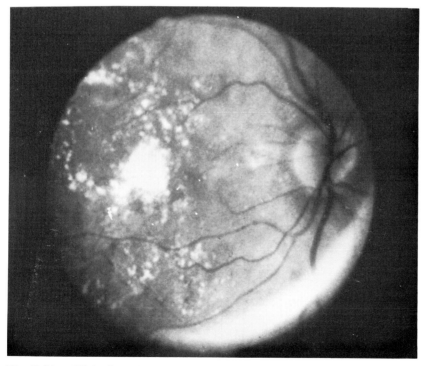

Fig. 9-5A. Diabetic retinopathy grade 1c with intraretinal edema involving the whole posterior pole. Visual acuity 20/400 (cf. Fig. 9-5B).

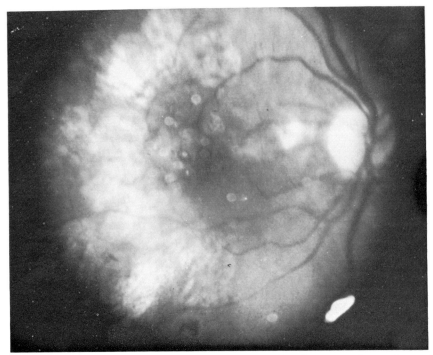

Fig. 9-5B. Same patient as Figure 9-5A, 6 months after argon laser photocoagulation to focal pathology. Visual acuity 20/200.

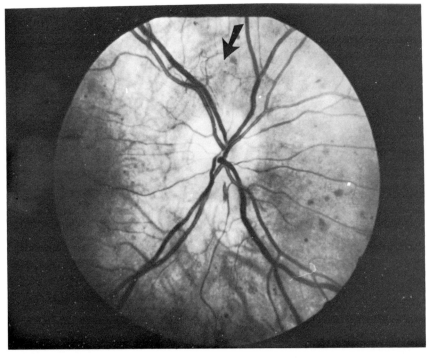

Fig. 9-6A. Diabetic retinopathy grade 2. There is an area of neovascularization in the plane of the retina immediately above the nerve head (arrow) (cf. Figs. 9-6B and 9-6C).

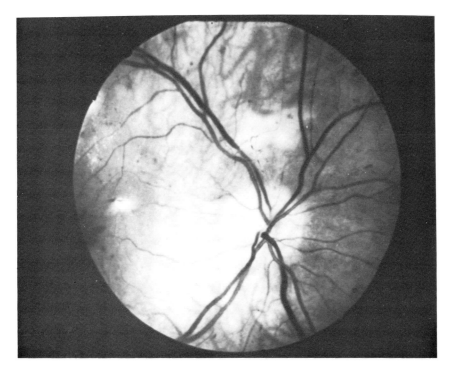

Fig. 9-6B. Same patient as in Figure 9-6A immediately after argon laser photocoagulation of the neovascular tuft (cf. Fig. 9-6C).

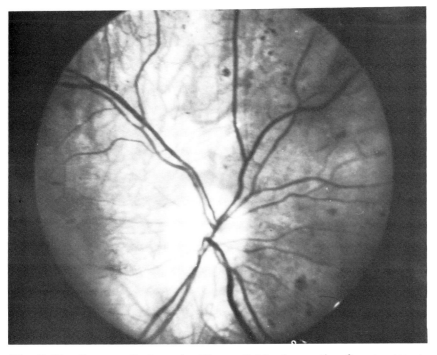

Fig. 9-6C. Same patient as in Figure 9-6A, 1 month after treatment.

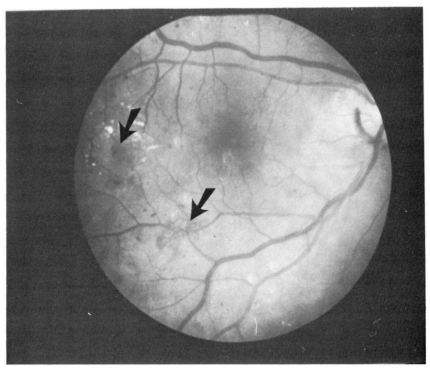

Fig. 9-7A. Diabetic retinopathy grade 2 with an area of neovascularization temporal from the macula and another inferotemporal from it with treatment with argon laser photocoagulation as indicated by arrows (cf. Fig. 9-7B).

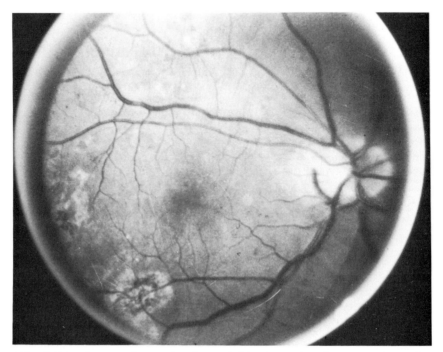

Fig. 9-7B. Same patient as in Figure 9-7A, 2 months after argon laser photocoagulation of the tufts.

second time to complete the destruction of the tuft. Figure 9-8A shows another area of neovascularization at the nasal edge of the macula. Hyperpigmentation is present 6 months after a single treatment had obliterated the tuft (Fig. 9-8B). Every attempt should be made to obliterate a tuft of neovascularization in the maculopapillar bundle in a single session. Repeated treatments almost certainly will give nerve fiber bundle field defects; a single treatment usually will not.

In grade 3 patients we originally used direct photocoagulation of the frond as shown in Figure 9-9A before treatment. The frond had just been coagulated in Figure 9-9B; it is hyperemic and tends to bleed. While this frond atrophied considerably 6 weeks later (Fig. 9-9C) without a nerve fiber bundle field defect, many like this bled after treatment. Approximately 15 to 20 percent of such cases had this complication. Dr. Little and I wondered if there were better ways to do this than by such a "frontal assault." We have been taking parallel routes in approaching these problems since March 1972; we will be comparing our results in 1974. As he discusses in Chapter 11, he is doing feeder vessel-frond coagulation and panretinal photocoagulation (PRP); I am not treating the nerve head at all, but doing only PRP. In PRP, 500-μ or 1000-μ exposures are placed from the nerve head to the equator, excepting the macula and the maculopapillar bundle. Figure 9-10A shows the nerve head and adjacent nasal retina of a patient with grade 3 diabetic retinopathy before treatment with PRP with argon laser photocoagulation. These lesions are contiguous 500 μ spot sizes going out along the vessels but avoiding the maculopapillar bundle. Figure 9-10B shows the patient immediately after treatment. Figure 9-10C shows the patient 3 weeks

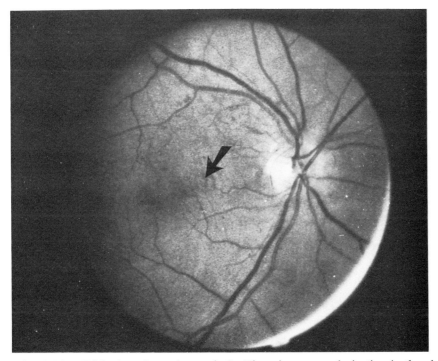

Fig. 9-8A. Diabetic retinopathy grade 2. There is neovascularization in the plane of the retina at the nasal macula on the maculopapillar bundle as indicated by arrow (cf. Fig. 9-8B).

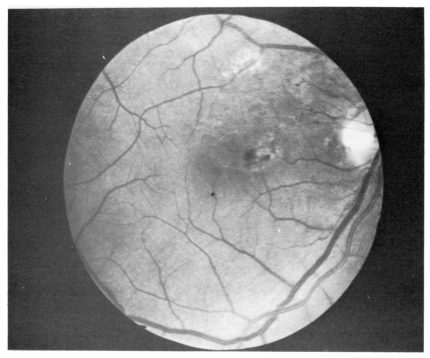

Fig. 9-8B. Same patient as in Figure 9-8A, 6 months after argon laser photo-coagulation performed in a single session. No nerve fiber bundle field defect is present.

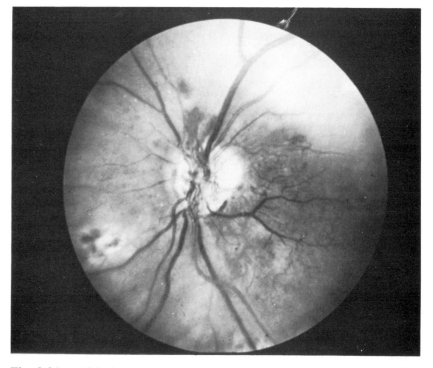

Fig. 9-9A. Diabetic retinopathy grade 3 immediately before treatment with argon laser photocoagulation (cf. Figs. 9-9B and 9-9C).

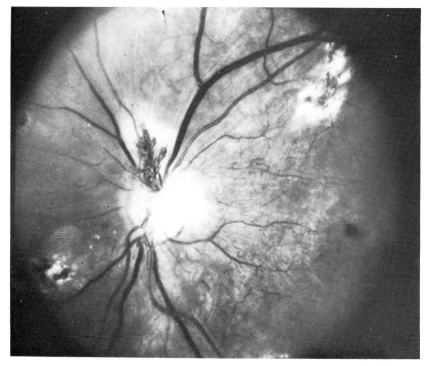

Fig. 9-9B. Same patient as in Figure 9-9A immediately after direct photocoagulation of the frond with argon laser photocoagulation (cf. Fig. 9-9C).

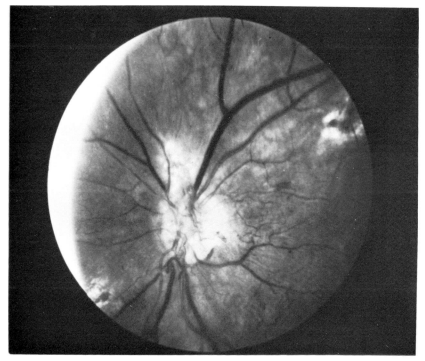

Fig. 9-9C. Same patient as in Figure 9-9A, 7 weeks after argon laser photocoagulation. The frond has atrophied considerably. No nerve fiber bundle field defect is present.

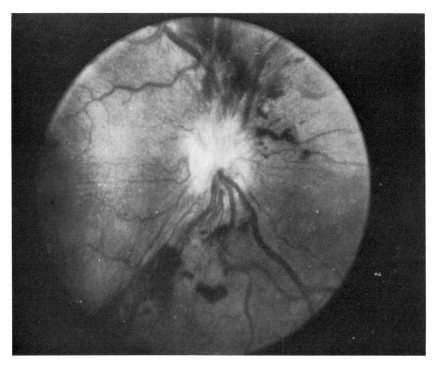

Fig. 9-10A. Diabetic retinopathy grade 3 before treatment by PRP technique using argon laser photocoagulation. The nerve head and adjacent nasal retina can be seen. Visual acuity 20/40 (cf. Figs. 9-10B and 9-10C).

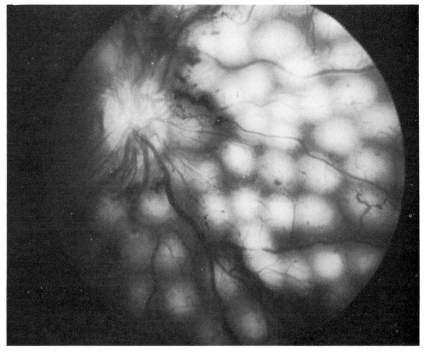

Fig. 9-10B. Same patient as in Figure 9-10A immediately after treatment by PRP technique using argon laser photocoagulation (cf. Fig. 9-10C).

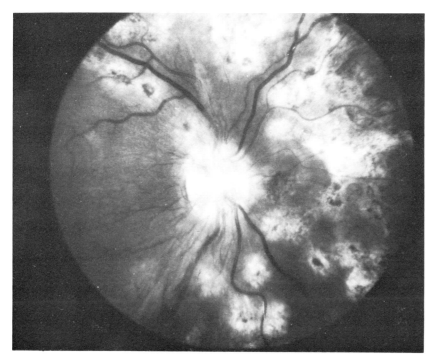

Fig. 9-10C.   Same patient as Figure 9-10A 3 weeks after PRP showing decongestion of the retina and decrease of nerve head neovascularization. Visual acuity 20/80 +1.

after treatment demonstrating a striking improvement in the appearance of the retina, especially the neovascularization on the nerve head and reduction of the caliber of the veins which were engorged pretreatment. Figure 9-11A shows the eye of a patient with a good deal of disc neovascularization. This patient had been treated with argon laser photocoagulation directly on the disc neovascularization at the site indicated by the arrow; then he was treated with PRP. Figure 9-11B shows the same patient 3 weeks after treatment with very little neovascularization left in the glial veil. He has some optic atrophy which I think is necessary for success with this technique. I think if the nerve head does not show some pallor, treatment has not been extensive enough. Such patients, typically, have some reduction of field noticeable at night; field reduction is about 20 degrees with a 2-mm white target at 1 meter.

The time, power, and spot size settings recommended for argon laser photocoagulation of various grades of diabetic retinopathy are shown in Table 9-2.

So, in summary, we have discussed and demonstrated with photographs the patients that we believe *should* be treated and our current thinking as to *how* they should be treated with argon laser slit-lamp photocoagulation.

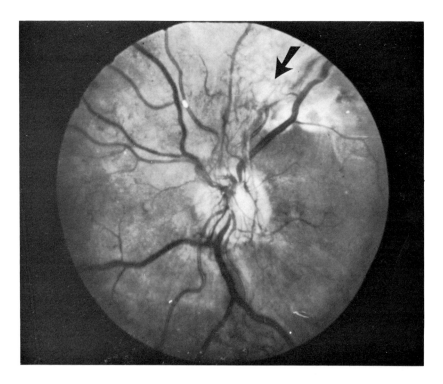

Fig. 9-11A. Diabetic retinopathy grade 3 before PRP. Neovascularization in the plane of the retina indicated by the arrow had previously been treated by argon laser photocoagulation (cf. Fig. 9-11B).

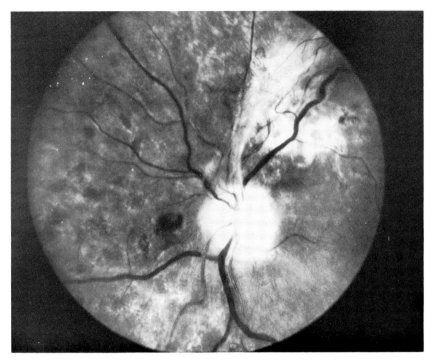

Fig. 9-11B. Same patient as Figure 9-11A 3 weeks after PRP had been completed. Note regression of neovascularization on the nerve head and reduction in the caliber of the retinal veins.

Table 9–2
Treatment Levels of Diabetic Retinopathy

Grade and Technique	Spot Size Diameter (μ)	Time (sec)	Power (mW)
1a focal (rarely treat)	50–200	0.05–0.2	100–300
1b focal	50–200	0.05–0.2	100–300
1c focal	100–200	0.05–0.5	100–500
2 frond	100–200	0.1–0.5	100–500
3 feeder vessel	50	0.1–0.5	100–250
3 frond	50	0.1–0.2	100–250
3 PRP	500–1000	0.05–0.2	500–1500
4 (rarely treat)	As grade 3, depending on modality used: focal, feeder-frond, and/or PRP		

Edward Okun

Chapter 10

Selection of Cases for Photocoagulation by Xenon or Argon

To begin with, I do not think there is any question as to what we are all trying to do, that is, to prolong the visual life of an eye with proliferative diabetic retinopathy. We know that these eyes lose vision primarily because of vitreous hemorrhage, fibrous proliferation, and traction detachments. If we can avoid vitreous hemorrhage and eliminate neovascular proliferation, we can protect many eyes from complete blindness; and if we can prevent the accumulation of edema and exudation in the macula before visual acuity has been irreversibly reduced, then we might be able to save those eyes destined for macular blindness. Initially [1] (from 1960 to 1963) we selected for treatment only patients who had had vitreous hemorrhages because we thought that the site of vitreous hemorrhagic activity, once coagulated, would not bleed again. We also learned that we could immediately stop the hemorrhagic process at that point. Immediately after photocoagulation, the blood turns pink, then white, and then disappears. Figure 10-1 shows the site of origination of a vitreous hemorrhage. This eye was photocoagulated, and 3.5 weeks later a scar has formed and the hemorrhage has disappeared (Fig. 10-2). Other areas in this eye were photocoagulated, the last treatment being in 1967. This patient still has good vision. When you see an eye that has had a preretinal hemorrhage of this type, you can rest assured that there is neovascularization present under the hemorrhage. These new vessels are usually eliminated with the treatment of the overlying blood. However, when the hemorrhage clears, there may be some neovascularization remaining. This should then be treated.

We next reasoned that it would be better to eliminate these areas before they have had a chance to bleed. The next series of figures illustrates a vitreous hemorrhage originating from such a zone. We did not photocoagulate the neovascular zone shown in Figure 10-3; the result is shown in Figure 10-4. At this stage, one can still photocoagulate the site of origination of the hemorrhage (Fig. 10-5); 3 weeks post photocoagulation (Fig. 10-6) the neovascularization has been eliminated and the hemorrhage has been absorbed.

* All figures in this chapter except Figs. 10-7, 10-8, and 10-9 appear in the color section.

Areas of neovascularization of the type shown in Figure 10-7 can bleed and can also grow. This particular one is growing, and a new zone of neovascularization is now starting (Fig. 10-8). It was photocoagulated with the xenon photocoagulator (Fig. 10-9); 4 months after treatment, the neovascularization has been replaced by a photocoagulation scar (Fig. 10-10). This patient has had a 5-year follow-up; there is 20/20 visual acuity in the left eye.

Sometimes neovascularization starts up very close to the macula; after it has grown, to eliminate it may force you to treat closer to the macula than you would like. So rather than wait, we elected to treat the case shown in Figure 10-11. This was about 6 years ago; the eye continues to do well (Fig. 10-12), with 20/25 visual acuity; the other eye is blind.

Next we come to slightly more advanced pathology (Fig. 10-13). These areas are difficult to eliminate, sometimes requiring a technique which combines

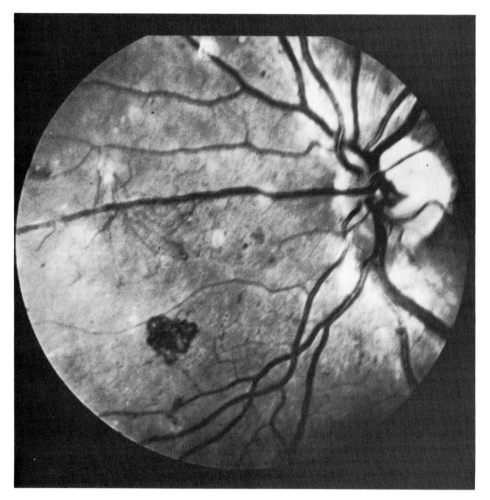

Fig. 10-7. Left eye of 23-year-old white male with diabetes of 15 years' duration. Fundus photograph shows nest of neovascular tissue two disc diameters inferonasal to the disc (cf. Figs. 10-8, 10-9, and 10-10).

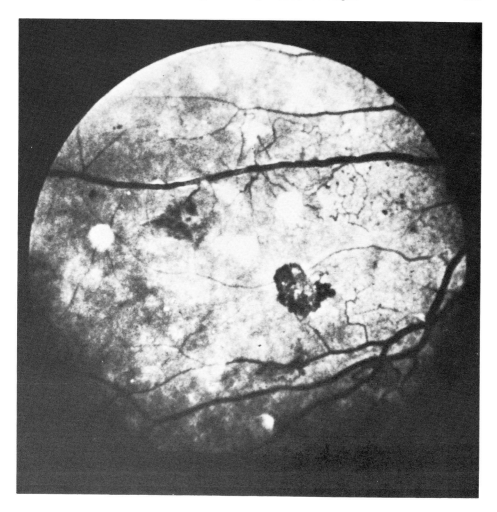

Fig. 10-8. Same patient as in Figure 10-7, 2 months later. Fundus photograph shows mulberry-like cluster of neovascularization two disc diameters inferonasal to the disc (*arrow*), an area of neovascularization along the course of the inferonasal vein below, and a zone of intraretinal microangiopathy above the lesion. The zone above the lesion has grown and behaves like neovascular tissue (cf. Figs. 10-9 and 10-10).

both xenon and argon. Xenon photocoagulation was used in this case (Fig. 10-14). The follow-up (Fig. 10-15) shows a few little fine vessels (better seen in stereo) remaining. One now has a choice of either treating with argon or waiting to see what these vessels do, because they frequently shrivel up over a matter of years of follow-up; however, if they begin to grow, I think they should be eliminated with the argon laser.

This patient (Fig. 10-16) had advanced pathology all over her eye. She was told that she might require a pituitary ablation, but that we would first try to treat the eye with photocoagulation. Large areas were photocoagulated (Fig. 10-17), and she presently has 2 years of follow-up. She still has 20/20 visual acuity in both eyes. We now have a series of 10 or 12 patients who fall into this

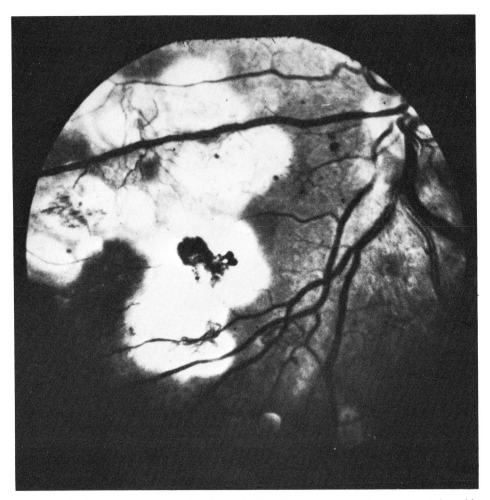

Fig. 10-9. Same patient as in Figure 10-7. Photocoagulation lesions are 1 day old. Note that the most intense lesions are placed directly over the angiomatous lesion (cf. Figs. 10-8 and 10-10).

category (termed rubeosis retinae by Meyer-Schwickerath) which requires really massive photocoagulation. Post-photocoagulation, the patients may tell you they have the sensation that they are looking through a tube; if you do a visual field, you can confirm the constricted visual field. But they are seeing; and quite frankly, I have not seen too many patients with this degree of pathology do any better with pituitary ablation, because these membranes show increasing fibrosis and retraction despite pituitary ablation. So it is a matter of exchanging a very scarred retina with macular function for one that would have gone on to vitreous hemorrhage and complete blindness.

Our approach is first to use xenon photocoagulation in every patient, because this is the safest means of photocoagulation.[2] Our xenon photocoagulation looks not too unlike that which Dr. Zweng showed us with argon photocoagulation (Chapter 9). I do not care if one wants to use the argon laser to do that. In our hands, it is simpler to perform initial widespread photocoagulation with the

4.5-degree spot-size xenon photocoagulator. Having had a great deal of experience with both xenon and argon laser techniques, I certainly do not think that xenon light does any more damage to the eye.

The patient in Figure 10-18A was treated fairly vigorously. Six weeks later much of the disc is dried up in exactly the same way as Dr. Zweng has shown after widespread argon laser treatment (Fig. 10-18B). I wish this happened every time, but unfortunately it does not. But I think that we should give it a chance to happen. I do not think that we have had nearly as good results by starting right off at the disc with argon laser treatment. The disc is treated with the argon laser only if there is regrowth from the disc following an adequate period of follow-up, which is between 3 and 6 months.

The eye in Figure 10-19, with a dense vitreous hemorrhage, cannot be treated at this stage. But if you put the patient at bed rest, either at home or in the hospital, within 2 days to 2 weeks there may be enough absorption of the hemorrhage that it becomes a candidate for photocoagulation (Fig. 10-20). Figure 10-21 shows the eye 1 day after photocoagulation treatment, and Figure 10-22, 1 year later. Unfortunately there is a nerve fiber bundle field defect secondary to the photocoagulation scarring on the nasal side. The other eye did not receive peripapillary treatment, but rather scattered focal treatment away from the disc. It is now the worse eye by virtue of uncontrolled disc proliferation.

Peripapillary xenon photocoagulation appears to benefit eyes with neovascularization originating from the disc and adjacent areas. Figure 10-23 shows new vessels arising from the disc and extending upward from it 3 weeks following peripapillary photocoagulation. Over the years, subsequent peripapillary photocoagulation treatments were required to contain this neovascular growth. Four years later the eye was almost completely free of neovascularization (Fig. 10-24); so, after successful xenon photocoagulation it looks not unlike an eye successfully treated by argon laser photocoagulation. Figure 10-25 shows another eye which has some neovascularization extending inferonasal to the disc. Figure 10-26, taken nine months later, reveals that there has been no regrowth. Looking at this last figure, one could not say that this was not successfully treated by the argon laser. Figure 10-27 shows an eye with venous engorgement and a tremendous amount of surface neovascularization. Two weeks after extensive xenon photocoagulation, most of the neovascularization has been eliminated and the veins are no longer distended (Fig. 10-28).

Figure 10-29 illustrates two points: (1) this eye has received too little photocoagulation to be of benefit for such advanced surface proliferation; at this stage it had been "unsuccessfully treated" elsewhere; (2) it is not yet too advanced to respond to more extensive xenon and/or argon photocoagulation. Figure 10-30 shows the same eye 7 months following both xenon and argon photocoagulation in one session. The surface neovascularization was treated with xenon, and the elevated vessels with the argon laser.

Continuous follow-up and retreatment when necessary is as important in the therapy of diabetic retinopathy as it is in the treatment of cancer. Figure 10-31 shows "breakaway" neovascularization. Regrowth of new vessels has taken place at the edge of an old scar. Figure 10-32 shows that the retreatment has eliminated this new growth before it has had a chance to grow larger, lift away from the retina, or bleed into the vitreous.

Macular edema responds well to photocoagulation. Figure 10-33 and 10-34 show one that was treated with the xenon photocoagulator, and the follow-up is shown in Figure 10-35; this is an eye that started off with 20/70-1 and presently has 20/50 visual acuity. We have over 100 eyes that look like this. Argon laser photocoagulation with spot sizes under 200 μ result in scars which are difficult to find, but more importantly, I find a significant amount of residual hemorrhagic and exudative activity. Argon lesions of 200-μ spot size look somewhat better. There is some pigment accumulation but the lesions are very tiny, and quite frankly, thus far, I have not been as pleased with the argon laser treatment of maculopathy as I have been with xenon photocoagulation.

Figures 10-36, 10-37, and 10-38 show the maculopathy before, immediately after, and 11 months after argon laser photocoagulation, respectively. The lesions produced with argon laser are more distinct immediately following treatment than 11 months later. Right now I prefer the 3-degree xenon lesions to the 200-μ spot-size slit-lamp argon laser lesion for the treatment of diabetic maculopathy; our results have been better with it.

Figure 10-39 shows a zone of bleeding from an area that is pulled out from a vein branch right into the vitreous; this is a perfect case for argon laser treatment. It has been cut off with the argon laser (Fig. 10-40); hopefully it would snap back into the vitreous. That is exactly what happened—it broke away and it's just a little wisp (Fig. 10-41); and after a 1-year follow-up there has been no further bleeding.

There are certain cases that I am sure get worse with argon laser treatment. The eye in Figure 10-42 has too much proliferation to handle with the argon laser. Figure 10-43 shows the results of acute treatment. In Figure 10-44 the big fibrous membrane has retracted. I am sorry I ever treated that patient.

So, in summary, I would like to state that our approach is to treat all patients with neovascularization or macular edema. I think that the xenon photocoagulator should be used initially because, in my hands at least, the complication rate is much lower than with argon. I really cannot remember a hemorrhage occurring on the table with the xenon photocoagulator. I think that the argon laser can eliminate certain residual areas of neovascularization that the xenon photocoagulator cannot, and should be reserved for that. However, I feel that the therapeutic dose that is required to really do the job with the argon laser is too close to the LD-50, or lethal dose (hemorrhage-inducing or visual-field-limiting). I cannot think of a single thing that I do in retinal surgery that causes as much apprehension as trying to permanently eliminate those tiny new vessels that are microns away from very large succulent ones. I therefore favor peripapillary and peripheral treatment first, followed by direct treatment only if the disc vessels are not favorably affected by the former.

REFERENCES

1. Okun E, Cibis PA: The role of photocoagulation in the therapy of proliferative diabetic retinopathy. Arch Ophthalmol 75:337, 1966

2. Okun E, Johnston GP, Boniuk I: Management of Diabetic Retinopathy; A Stereoscopic Presentation. St. Louis, Mosby, 1971, p 68

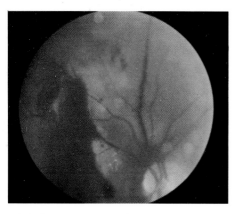 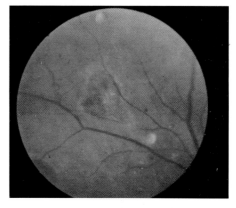

Fig. 10-1. (left) Left eye of 58-year-old white male with diabetes of 4 years' known duration. Vitreous hemorrhage originating from neovascularization just below superonasal arteriole. **Fig. 10-2. (right)** Same patient as in Figure 10-1, 3.5 weeks after photocoagulation scarring. Photocoagulation treatment had been directed to the site of origination of the vitreous hemorrhage.

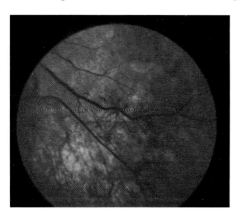 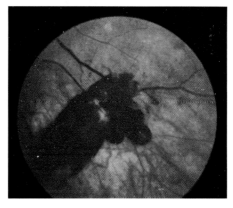

Fig. 10-3. (left) Right eye of a 43-year-old white female with diabetes of 22 years' duration. Twigs of neovascularization originate from the inferonasal venule. **Fig. 10-4. (right)** Same patient as in Figure 10-3, untreated, 5.5 months later. Vitreous hemorrhage originates from the zone of neovascularization.

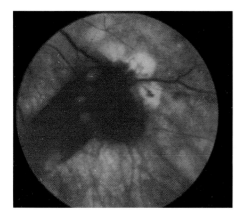 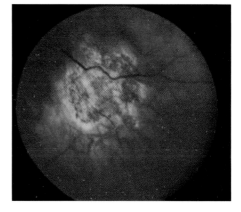

Fig. 10-5. (left) Same patient as in Figure 10-3, 10 minutes following photocoagulation treatment. Acute photocoagulation lesions cover areas of bare neovascularization as well as the zone of preretinal hemorrhage. Note the photocoagulation effects directly on the preretinal blood. **Fig. 10-6 (right)** Same patient as in Figure 10-3, 3 weeks later, showing elimination of neovascularization as well as absorption of hemorrhage. The inferonasal arteriole shows markedly decreased caliber.

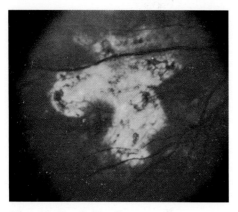 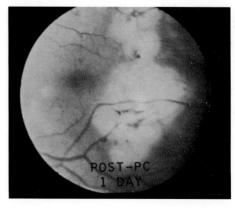

Fig. 10-10. (left) Same patient as in Figure 10-7. The same zone is shown approximately 4 months after photocoagulation. Neovascularization has been replaced by a photocoagulation scar. **Fig. 10-11. (right)** Left eye of 53-year-old white female with diabetes of 4 years' known duration. Twigs of neovascularization are present, temporal to the macula. This is one day following photocoagulation.

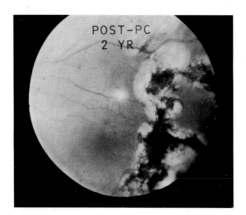 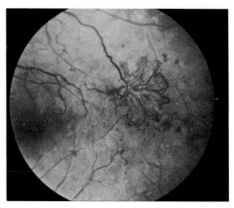

Fig. 10-12. (left) Same patient as in Figure 10-11, 2 years following photocoagulation. Visual acuity remains at 20/25+3. Note that photocoagulation scar has replaced neovascularization. **Fig. 10-13. (right)** Left eye of a 27-year-old white female with diabetes of 14 years' duration. Fundus photograph shows a fan of neovascularization superotemporal to the macula.

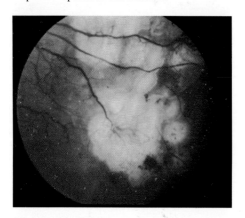 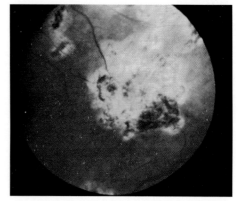

Fig. 10-14. (left) Appearance of 3-day-old photocoagulation lesions that surround the partially collapsed fan as well as confluent lesions along a superior branch of the superotemporal vein (cf. Figs. 10-13 and 10-15). **Fig. 10-15. (right)** One year following photocoagulation, several small atrophic twigs of surface neovascularization remain. Visual acuity in the eye remains at 20/25.

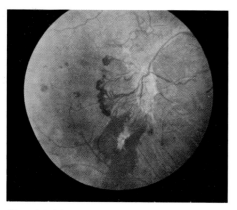 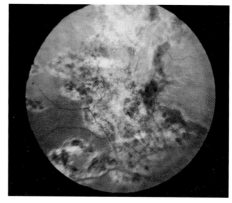

Fig. 10-16. (left) Right eye of juvenile diabetic showing advanced cartwheel neovascularization, early fibrosis, and vitreous hemorrhage. **Fig. 10-17. (right)** Same patient as in Figure 10-16, 6 months later, showing photocoagulation scar replacing neovascular zone.

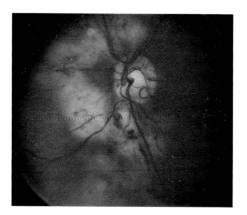 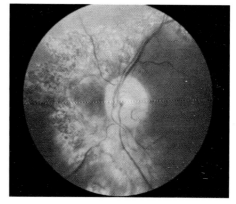

Fig. 10-18.A (left) Left eye of 50-year-old diabetic 1 day after photocoagulation of peripapillary neovascularization. **Fig. 10-18B. (right)** Same patient as in Figure 10-18A, 6 weeks later, showing elimination of peripapillary disc neovascularization.

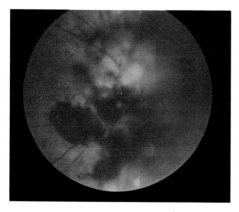 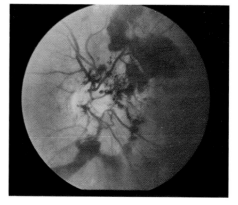

Fig. 10-19. (left) Dense vitreous hemorrhage which prevents photocoagulation (cf. Figs. 10-20, 10-21 and 10-22). **Fig. 10-20. (right)** Pre-treatment appearance after vitreous hemorrhage has cleared in eye with advanced disc and peripapillary neovascularization.

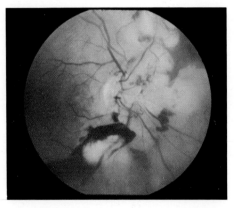 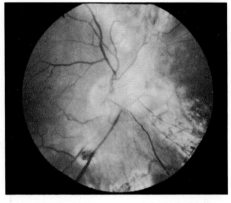

Fig. 10-21. (left) Same eye as in Figure 10-20, 1 day after photocoagulation treatment.
Fig. 10-22. (right) Same eye as in Figures 10-19, 10-20, and 10-21, 1 year later.

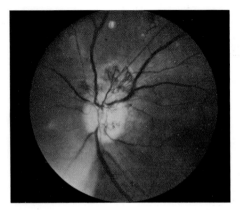 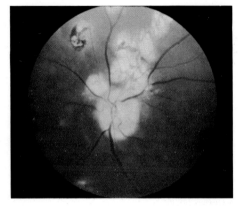

Fig. 10-23. (left) Residual disc and peripapillary neovascularization 3 weeks after peripapillary photocoagulation. **Fig. 10-24. (right)** Same eye as in Figure 10-23, 4 years later. Neovascularization of disc has dried up after additional treatment.

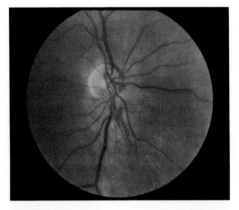 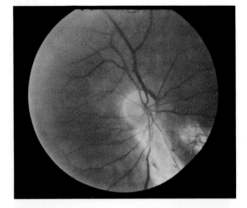

Fig. 10-25. (left) Neovascularization extends inferonasal to the disc. **Fig. 10-26. (right)** Same eye as in Figure 10-25, 9 months later showing elimination of disc and peripapillary neovascularization by peripapillary photocoagulation.

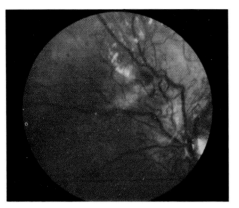 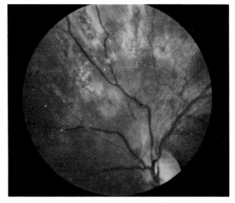

Fig. 10-27. (left) Left eye of 23-year-old white male with diabetes of 11 years' duration. Fundus photograph shows marked dilation of veins and surface neovascularization. **Fig. 10-28. (right)** Same patient as in Figure 10-27, 2 weeks after photocoagulation scarring. The photograph illustrates retinal elimination of most neovascularization. and marked decrease in the caliber of veins.

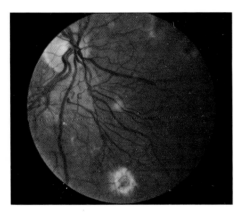 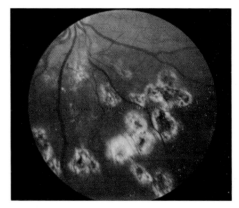

Fig. 10-29. (left) Fundus of juvenile diabetic after insufficient xenon photocoagulation. **Fig. 10-30. (right)** Same eye as in Figure 10-29, 7 months after combination xenon and argon laser photocoagulation. Most neovascularization has been eliminated.

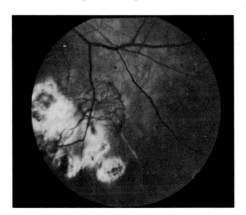 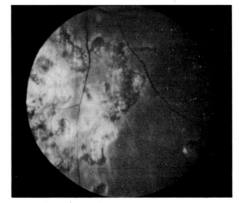

Fig. 10-31. (left) Left eye of 36-year-old white male with diabetes of 26 years' duration. "Breakaway" neovascularization extends across the inferior venule. Previous photocoagulation was done 2 years earlier. **Fig. 10-32. (right)** Same patient as in Figure 10-31, 2 months after coagulation. Neovascular fan has been eliminated by new photocoagulation scar.

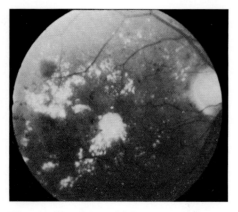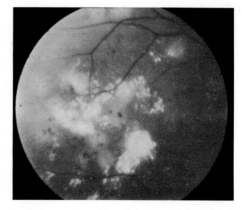

Fig. 10-33. (left) Right eye of 54-year-old while male with diabetes of 3 years'
known duration. Fundus photograph showing macular edema, hard yellow waxy exudates, and multiple zones of retinal microangiopathy. Visual acuity 20/70–1.
Fig. 10-34. (right) Same patient as in Figure 10-33, approximately 1 day following
photocoagulation. Photocoagulation lesions are directed to the areas of microangiopathy.

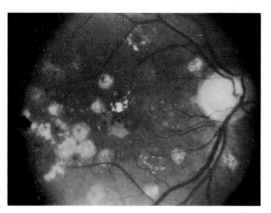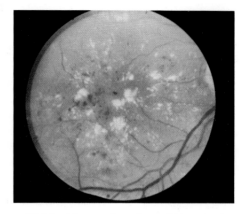

Fig. 10-35. (left) Same patient as in Figure 10-33, 15 months after photocoagulation. Marked resolution of the macular edema and absorption of hard waxy exudates
with replacement by fine photocoagulation scars. Visual acuity 20/50. **Fig. 10-36.
(right)** Fundus photograph shows exudative maculopathy.

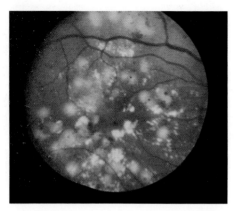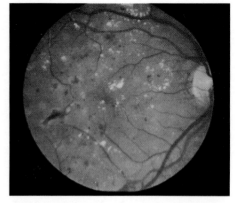

Fig. 10-37. (left) Same eye as in Figure 10-36, immediately after argon laser photocoagulation. **Fig. 10-38. (right)** Same eye as in Figure 10-36, 11 months later.

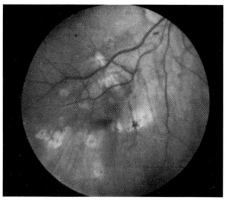 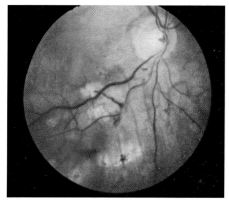

Fig. 10-39. (left) Vitreous hemorrhage secondary to traction on a small new vessel.
Fig. 10-40. (right) Same eye as in Figure 10-39, 1 day after argon laser photocoagulation treatment.

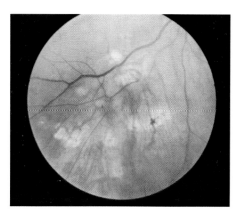 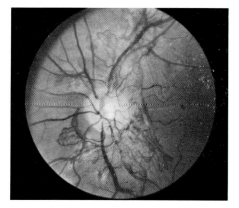

Fig. 10-41. (left) Same eye as in Figure 10-39, 2 months after treatment. New vessel has been severed from its vein of origination and vitreous hemorrhage has cleared.
Fig. 10-42. (right) Very large neovascular membrane covers disc and approximately five disc diameters of posterior pole.

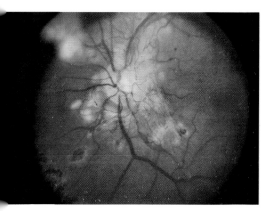 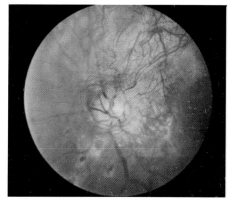

Fig. 10-43. (left) Same eye as in Figure 10-42, 1 day after argon laser photocoagulation. Most vessels have been occluded. **Fig. 10-44. (right)** Same eye as in Figure 10-42, 3 months later. Membrane has opacified and retracted with regrowth of vessels.

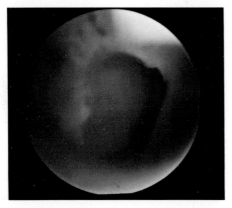 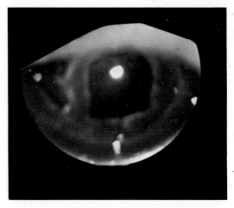

Fig. 14-12. (left) Fundus view through a hole cut in an intravitreal membrane with the vitrophage. **Fig. 14-13. (right)** Photograph showing a hole cut in an intravitreal membrane behind the pupil.

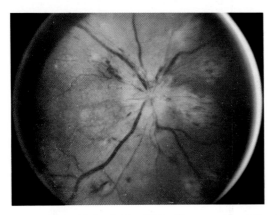 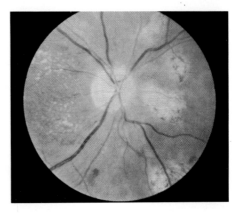

Fig. 21-3. (left) This 23-year-old white female has had diabetes for 14 years. At the time of this photograph the patient was 4 months' pregnant, and a massive congestion of the vessels on the optic disc can be seen, as well as early neovascularization and pronounced venous congestion. **Fig. 21-4. (right)** Same patient as in Fig. 21-3. Six weeks following a therapeutic abortion, the optic disc and vessels in the posterior pole have returned to an approximately normal appearance, but small round hemorrhages are still present in the paramacular region and a thread of neovascularization is present in the inferotemporal quadrant of the optic disc.

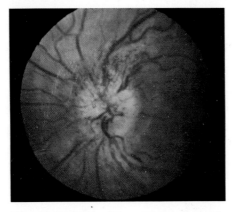 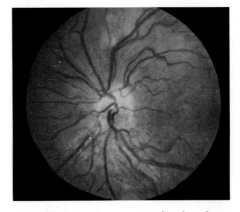

Fig. 21-5. (left) Disc neovascularization and papilledema in eye previously photocoagulated. **Fig. 21-6. (right)** Same eye as in Fig. 21-5, 3 months after patient had been treated for congestive cardiac failure.

Hunter L. Little

Chapter 11

Retinal Neovascularization in Diabetes Mellitus and the Role of Fluorescein Angiography in Argon Laser Photocoagulation

Michaelson postulated that hypoxia plays a significant role in stimulating the growth of retinal vessels.[1] His conclusion resulted from extensive studies of fetal retinae of mice, cat, and man, in which he noted that capillary proliferation always occurred from the venules and that capillary growth was absent around arterioles. Ashton and Patz have shown independently the effect of elevated oxygen concentration on inhibiting the growth of immature retinal vessels in cats.[2,3] There are at least a dozen disease entities seen in the practice of ophthalmology which are associated with retinal neovascularization. These are discussed in our book, *Laser Photocoagulation and Fluorescein Angiography* (Table 11-1).[4] Some are covered in Chapter 8 by Dr. Morton Goldberg. Wise observed that retinal hypoxia was the underlying common denominator in all these disease

Table 11-1
Retinal Neovascularization

1. Diabetes mellitus
2. Central retinal vein occlusion
3. Hypertension
4. Eales's disease
5. Sickle cell anemia
6. Malaria
7. Pulseless disease
8. Radiation retinopathy
9. Polycythemia
10. Dysproteinemia (macroglobulinemia and cryoglobulinemia)
11. Coats' disease
12. Retrolental fibroplasia

states.[5] Retinal hypoxia is caused by impaired circulation or perfusion due to changes in blood content, blood flow, or blood vessels.

This presentation is restricted to retinal neovascularization in diabetes and to its management with argon laser photocoagulation. Some of the material was presented earlier this year in Ghent, Belgium.[6-8] The importance of high-speed fluorescein angiography in detecting feeder vessels to neovascular fronds is stressed in relation to treatment of proliferative diabetic retinopathy with argon laser photocoagulation. All patients are worked up very extensively; retinal drawings and photographs are done. The retinal evaluation includes all modalities using direct ophthalmoscopy, indirect ophthalmoscopy, and the slit-lamp biomicroscopic examination. Drawings in some respects are better than photographs because greater attention is required of the ophthalmologist to sketch the retina than to photograph it. Both sketches and photographs are essential. Red-free photography is also helpful in the work-up of the patient. The retinal vessels stand out much more vividly with red-free light than with ordinary white light. Patients should be photographed in this manner before getting fluorescein studies.

The patient's fixation point should be identified before treatment. This can be done with the fixation target on the camera, and with the argon laser aiming beam. The operator should have the patient fixate on the aiming light before beginning treatment; thus, this area can then be identified and avoided.

Because blood selectively absorbs argon laser radiation, immediate vascular occlusion is produced with immediate alteration in the hemodynamics. For this reason, argon laser photocoagulation is more dangerous than xenon arc photocoagulation. Argon laser retinal photocoagulation is microvascular surgery. It requires precise identification and accurate recognition of the direction of blood flow in the vessels to be treated. Occlusion of a venule or efferent vessel causes congestion and hemorrhage, whereas occlusion of an arteriole or afferent or feeder vessel enables one to treat neovascular fronds with much less risk of hemorrhage. Thus, fluorescein angiography is essential in retinal vascular diseases requiring photocoagulation. The importance of high resolution and high magnification of fluorescein angiograms in argon laser photocoagulation of proliferative retinopathy cannot be overstressed.

In addition to getting fluorescein angiograms, one sometimes injects fluorescein at the time of treatment. This is recommended in the nonproliferative diabetic retinopathy and in macular degenerative diseases. When treating a microaneurysm, many times adjacent microaneurysms not previously identified will fluoresce due to the activation of the fluorescein by the wavelength of the argon laser. Furthermore, a number of blot hemorrhages, which do not fluoresce on the angiogram, will fluoresce when treated. Thus, intravenous injection of fluorescein immediately before treatment is helpful in treating macular leaks.

Patz first demonstrated with fluorescein angiography the ability to identify feeder vessels to neovascular fronds.[9] This technique has been a tremendous help in reducing the number of hemorrhagic complications. Enlargements of the angiograms improve visualization of the feeder vessels. Another method suggested by Patz is to project the negative of the angiogram onto a screen. In the negative, the area of fluorescence is black rather than white (Fig. 11-1). Stereo angiography is another aid in visualizing feeder vessels.

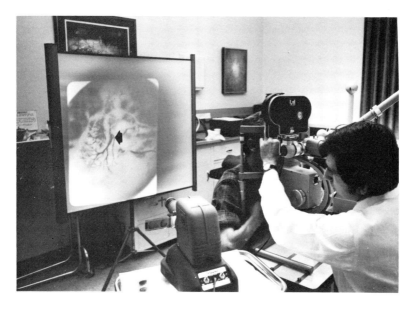

Fig. 11-1. Negative projection of fluorescein angiogram shows feeder vessel in black.

A common finding on fluorescein angiography is the presence of an avascular area of nonperfusion surrounding the distal margins of neovascularization. These areas of nonperfusion probably represent hypoxic but viable retina associated with the stimulus for retinal neovascularization. One should also treat the surrounding hypoxic areas as well as the abnormal vessels to eliminate and destroy that portion of the retina.

I would like to relate some of the experiences that we initially had in the feeder vessel technique. A young 22-year-old diabetic with proliferative retinopathy off the disc shows the early arterial phase of the angiogram (Fig. 11-2). There is early lamellar flow in the fluorescein study. This figure shows the feeder vessel coming off the disc. Argon laser photocoagulation was directed only to the feeder vessel. One day following treatment to the feeder vessel, only the vascular frond is markedly reduced, showing just a little fluorescence in some areas but absence in others (Fig. 11-3). Unfortunately this patient developed a much greater proliferation of vessels with subsequent hemorrhage and blindness.

Figure 11-4 illustrates the importance of fluorescein angiography in identifying feeder vessels in the optic disc. On the arterial phase of the angiogram, the veins are completely black, and the feeder vessel is fluorescing before the dye reaches the frond. This particular vessel, which looked like a venule because of its engorged dark appearance, rather than an arteriole, is actually an afferent vessel (Fig. 11-5). The feeder vessel was treated without treating the frond. After the treatment of this vessel, fluorescein no longer reached the frond (Fig. 11-6). There is increased fluorescence at the site treated because of damage to the vessel, causing increased perfusion at that point. There is nonperfusion of the vessel distal to the point of treatment. Blood is segmented in a fork of the treated vessel.

Another example showing the feeder vessel technique is illustrated in Figures 11-7 and 11-8. This patient has proliferative retinopathy of the disc. In the early

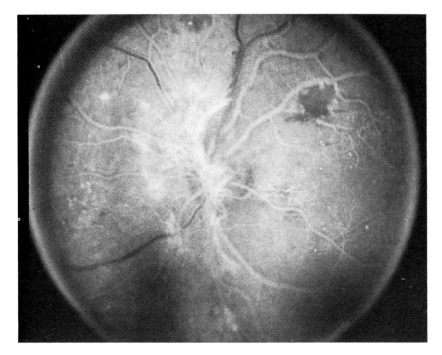

Fig. 11-2. Pretreatment angiogram of patient with proliferative diabetic retinopathy (cf. Fig. 11-3).

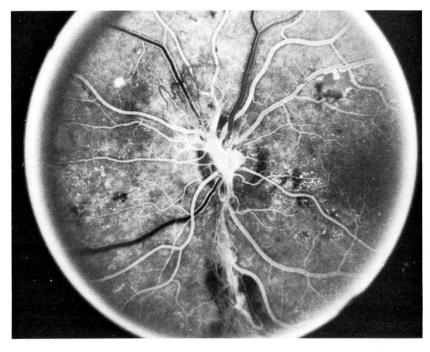

Fig. 11-3. One day post treatment of feeder vessel shows only nonfilling of neovascular frond (cf. Fig. 11-2).

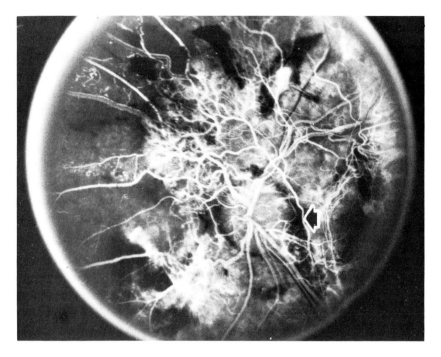

Fig. 11-4. Large vessel resembling a vein which proves to be a feeder vessel on angiography (cf. Figs. 11-5 and 11-6).

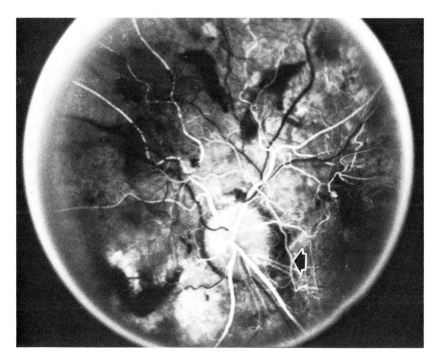

Fig. 11-5. Arterial phase of angiogram identifying afferent vessel (cf. Figs. 11-4 and 11-6).

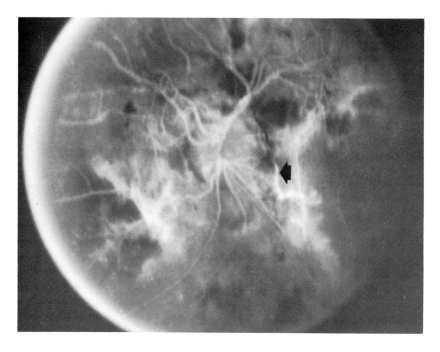

Fig. 11-6. Nonfilling of frond distal to point where feeder vessel was coagulated (cf. Figs. 11-4 and 11-5).

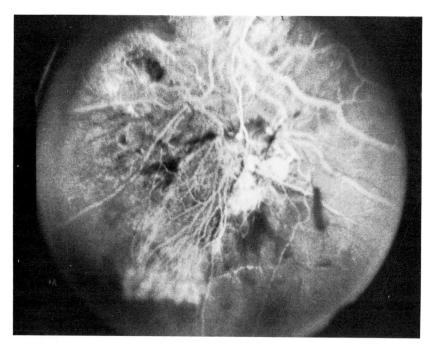

Fig. 11-7. Angiogram shows large juxtapapillary neovascular frond (cf. Fig. 11-8).

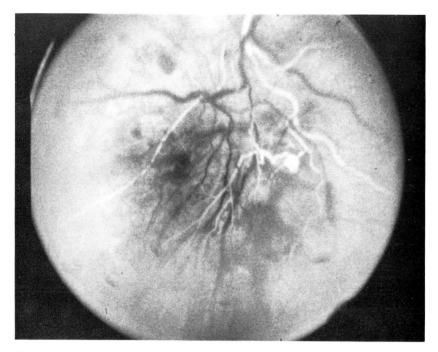

Fig. 11-8. Arterial phase of angiogram shows dark large venous channels unfilled with fluorescein. These are avoided in the initial stage of treatment (cf. Fig. 11-7).

angiogram of this same case, one cannot identify the feeder vessel, but one can see large dark vessels that are efferent vessels which should be avoided in the treatment (Fig. 11-8). Treatment is directed to the suspected feeder vessels, coming off the inferotemporal branch. Once the feeder vessel is treated, then photocoagulation of the entire frond is done with less likelihood of hemorrhage. Before using the feeder vessel technique there were a number of hemorrhagic complications resulting from coagulation of the entire frond without first obliterating the feeder vessel. After 1 year the visual acuity is 20/20, and there has not been recurrence of the proliferative retinopathy. There is pallor on the disc. In order to achieve quiescence of the retinopathy, extensive photocoagulation is necessary, which usually results in pallor of the optic nerve head.

Another case illustrates proliferative diabetic retinopathy in a juvenile diabetic with the vessels extending off the disc into the vitreous (Figs. 11-9 and 11-10). The feeder vessel is identified off the optic disc. After closure of its feeder vessel, the entire frond was treated. Fluorescein angiography shows that the area of fluorescence is markedly reduced. There is a small residual frond which was treated subsequently. After 1 year no recurrent neovascularization has occurred (Fig. 11-11). The latter angiogram was taken in the full venous phase to compare with the pretreatment angiogram.

Disc neovascularization frequently presents an "I" pattern (Fig. 11-12) of neovascularization. Following treatment there is reduced leakage, but 6 months later there is marked recurrent proliferation of vessels (Fig. 11-13). The feeder vessel was identified and treated; subsequently the whole frond was coagulated which resulted in marked obliteration of the vessels. The eye looked absolutely

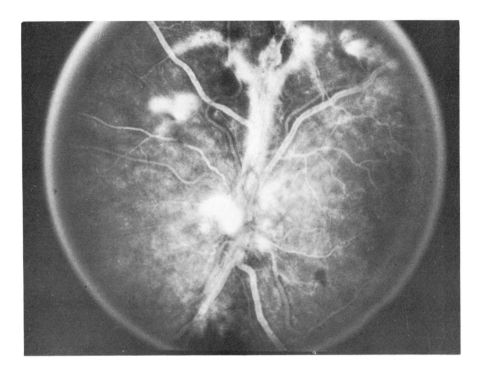

Fig. 11-9.   Large neovascular frond in juvenile diabetic (cf. Figs. 11-10 and 11-11).

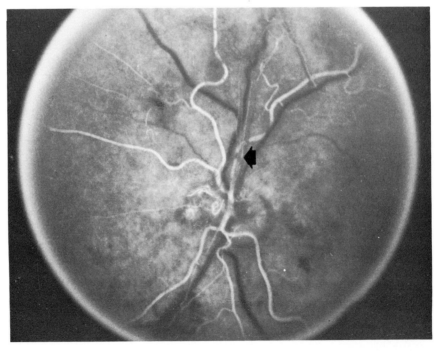

Fig. 11-10.   Arterial phase of angiogram identifies feeder vessel (cf. Figs. 11-9 and 11-11).

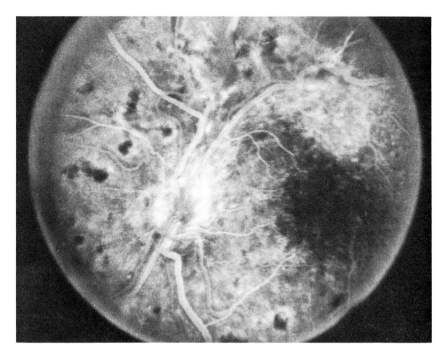

Fig. 11-11. One year post treatment shows no recurrent neovascularization (cf. Figs. 11-9 and 11-10).

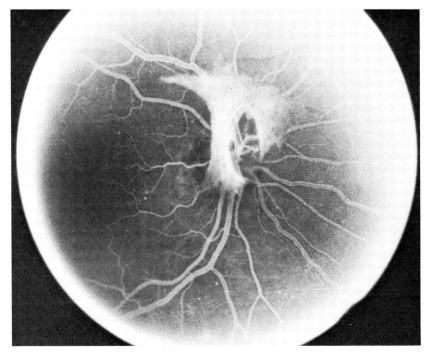

Fig. 11-12. Pretreatment angiogram of proliferative diabetic retinopathy (cf. Fig. 11-13).

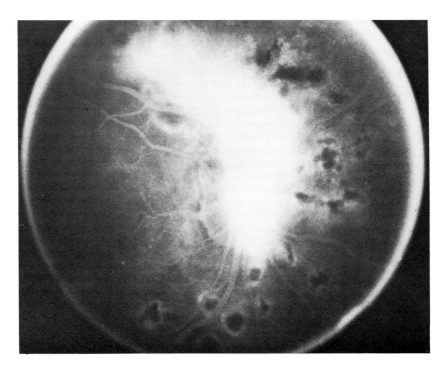

Fig. 11-13. Recurrent neovascularization 6 months after initial photocoagulation (cf. Fig. 11-12).

fantastic, but within the next 6 weeks it bled from a recurrent vessel. These patients are seldom completely well. One must continue to follow them closely. Follow-up examinations are advisable each 2 to 3 months. This point is illustrated below.

Since 36 percent of cases treated with the feeder vessel technique show recurrent growth of vessels, in July 1971 a combination of feeder vessel and frond treatment with pan-retinal photocoagulation was begun. Aiello and Beetham, and Wessing and Meyer-Schweigerath have independently recommended multiple 360-degree application of treatment in an attempt to reduce the stimulus of neovascularization.[10-11] First one treats the feeder and the frond, then pan-retinal photocoagulation is performed over 360 degrees. To be effective, at least 800 to 1200 lesions are required, in addition to those placed directly on the neovascular frond. The usual instrument settings for pan-retinal photocoagulation are as follows: 500-μ spot, 400 to 500 mW at 0.1 seconds in the paramacular and peripapillary area, and 1000 μ, 800 to 1000 mW at 0.1 seconds for midperipheral and peripheral lesions. The macula and maculopapular bundle are not included in panretinal photocoagulation.

Follow-up studies are grouped into the following three categories: (1) those with photocoagulation to the frond, (2) feeder-vessel treatment combined with photocoagulation of frond, and (3) feeder-vessel and frond treatment combined with pan-retinal photocoagulation (Table 11-2). The first group of 50 eyes with proliferative diabetic retinopathy treated without feeder technique were followed from 4 to 12 months. Sixty percent were better and 22 percent were worse; 12 percent remained the same. How many actually reached the stage of quiescence? That is the objective in the treatment of diabetic retinopathy. If one treats an area of

Table 11-2

Argon Laser Photocoagulation of Proliferative Diabetic Retinopathy
(4-to- 12-month follow-up)

	Frond Alone	Feeder Plus Frond	Feeder Plus 360
No. eyes	50	28	41
Better (%)	60	79	88
Same (%)	12	—	—
Worse (%)	22	13	13
Quiescent (%)	12	7	55
Hemorrhage (%)	16	6	5

neovascularization at 12 o'clock but a second frond at 3 o'clock is not eliminated, one still has vessels. The patient is better because he has only one frond rather than two, but the danger of losing the eye from hemorrhage is still present. Only 12 percent in this group reached the end point of quiescence that you wish to achieve at treatment. Twelve percent had significant hemorrhage, that is, hemorrhages which interfere with vision or which alter ability to treat the patient.

With the feeder vessel and frond treatment in 28 cases of proliferative diabetic retinopathy, 79 percent rather than 60 percent were better; however, only 7 were quiescent. If one takes the 41 eyes treated by the combined feeder and frond with pan-retinal photocoagulation, 88 percent were better and 55 percent were quiescent after 4 to 12 months.

In the feeder-frond treatment group, one initially reduces vascularization but the fronds recur. Many of them are probably worse than they would have been if we had left them alone. On the other hand, with combined feeder-frond treatment plus 360-degree ablation, 55 percent of the patients are now quiescent. The incidence of hemorrhage is 5 percent, which is less than the 16 percent that occurs with nonfeeder coagulation.

In conclusion, the best current method to treat proliferative diabetic retinopathy seems to be the use of feeder and frond coagulation combined with 360-degree pan-retinal photocoagulation. It is too early to make any conclusions, but obviously the initial results are much better at this time of follow-up with this technique than with the other methods of treatment. Probably the safest technique is first to perform panretinal photocoagulation in 3 sessions over a 7 to 10 day period followed 4 weeks later by feeder-frond photocoagulation of the residual neovascular areas.

REFERENCES

1. Michaelson IC: The mode of development of the vascular system at the retina, with some observations on its significance for certain retinal diseases. Trans Ophthalmol Soc UK 68:137–180, 1949

2. Ashton N: Oxygen and the growth and development of retinal vessels. In vivo and in vitro studies. Am J Ophthalmol 62:412–435, 1966

3. Patz A: The role of oxygen in retrolental fibroplasia. Trans Am Ophthalmol Soc 66:940–985, 1968

4. Zweng HC, Little HL and Peabody RR: Laser Photocoagulation and Fluorescein Angiography. St. Louis, Mosby, p 176

5. Wise GN: Retinal neovascularization. Trans Am Ophthalmol Soc 54:729–826, 1956

6. Little HL: Argon laser retinal photo-coagulation instrumentation and general techniques. In Symposium on Light Coagulation, Univ. Ghent 1972. Williams & Wilkins, 1973, p 17–26

7. Little HL: Argon laser therapy of diabetic retinopathy. In Symposium on Light Coagulation, Univ. Ghent 1972. Williams & Wilkins, 1973, p 77–84

8. Little HL: Prevention complications in argon laser retinal photocoagulation. In Symposium on Light Coagulation, Univ. Ghent 1972. Williams & Wilkins, 1973, p 87–95

9. Patz A: A guide to argon laser photo-coagulation. Sur Ophthalmol 16 (No. 4):249–257, 1972

10. Aiello LM, Beetham WD, et al: Ruby laser photocoagulation in treatment of diabetic proliferative retinopathy: preliminary report, in Goldberg MF, Fine SL (ed): Symposium on Treatment of Diabetic Retinopathy. US Public Health Service Publ 1890, Washington, 1969, pp 437–463

11. Wessing, AK, Meyer-Schwickerath G: Results of photocoagulation in diabetic retinopathy, in Goldberg MF, Fine SL (eds): Symposium on Treatment of Diabetic Retinopathy. US Public Health Service Publ 1890, Washington, 1969, pp 569–592

Francis L'Esperance

Chapter 12
Argon Laser Photocoagulation in Diabetic Lesions

I would like to address my remarks to the treatment of proliferative retinopathy and particularly to neovascularization of the disc itself. During the past 56 months, since the inception of argon laser photocoagulation, we have had the opportunity to treat 2400 to 2500 cases of diabetic retinopathy with the argon laser. Next week, 2160 of these cases will be reported at the Academy; they had retinal-vitreal neovascularization, extending either from the retina itself or from the disc into the vitreous body. Argon laser photocoagulation, as has so nicely been pointed out by the previous speakers, is quite similar to xenon arc photocoagulation. There is a difference, however. The xenon arc, as you know, has the full spectrum from 4,000 to 16,000 Å, including the infrared component. The argon laser has anywhere from six to eight wavelengths, depending upon the power output. The primary wavelengths are at the 4880Å line and also the 5145Å line. These are absorbed very highly by blood and converted to heat with direct coagulation to the surface of the blood component. When penetration is needed, such as in malignant melanomas, areas of thick glial proliferation, and areas of preretinal blood, as Dr. Okun pointed out (Chapter 10), the xenon arc may, for some reasons, be better than the argon. This is primarily because of the xenon arc infrared component which has the definite advantage of having greater penetration. Also, according to the remarks of Dr. Goldberg (Chapter 8), the argon beam as it strikes a vessel, will create heat on the surface of the blood vessel which radiates into the perivascular area. This is one of the difficulties—and special techniques have to be employed, as you will see here—for the obliteration of high flow vessels such as the main arterioles. But for the most part, argon laser photocoagulation, at least in the first four instances, functions much as the xenon arc. You can cause ablation of the retina, the obliteration of hemorrhagic sites, the destruction of peripheral neovascularization, and the production of the chorioretinal adhesions. This happens with either the xenon, the argon, the krypton, of the yttrium-aluminum-argon (YAG) laser, or any type of laser that you use, other than those lasers operating in the infrared part of the spectrum.

Because you can produce a 50-μ spot beam, you can approach the fovea within 150 or so microns and coagulate an angioma or a leakage area. You cannot do this with the xenon arc without the threat of striae or some other type of distortion of the foveal region. Obliteration of the peri- and epipapillary neovascularization, which is our discussion today, is also the sole province of the argon laser simply because the blood is acting as its own absorption site and it is converting the blue-green wavelengths into heat. With the xenon arc, for instance, only 25 percent of the wavelengths are in the highly absorbed blue end of the spectrum and, therefore, a large amount of energy has to enter the eye to produce a similar result. Also, the fact that you cannot focus the xenon as small as the argon makes the argon far superior for this type of work. Microplumbing techniques, I think, will be of great use in the future. Many things have to be worked out with the eventual capability of being able to measure the pressure in the chorioretinal vasculature in order to illustrate or demonstrate flow patterns in the eyes, either by television or through the wide-angle Nikon camera. In these areas, where the abnormal flow mechanisms, hemodynamics, and the pressure gradients can be tabulated for each individual patient, hopefully at some time, a coagulation technique can be devised to counteract the defective process.

For the purpose of the presentation at the Academy meeting, I have divided, over the course of the last 56 months, the neovascularization extending into the vitreous into five types. I divided these because they do differ in their growth characteristics, and they differ in their hazards as far as argon laser photocoagulation is concerned. They differ in the technique required and also in the type of devastation that they can cause in an eye. So, at least from a photocoagulation viewpoint, the five types of neovascularization will be described. This is epipapillary neovascularization that extends a short distance above the optic nerve toward the vitreous (Fig. 12-1). The areas of neovascularization are extremely fibrillar and thread-like. They carry very little hemoglobin and therefore are extremely difficult to photocoagulate. They usually do not extend along any of the arcades at this early stage. They probably are an early stage of what I call the papillovitreal type of neovascularization that we will see later (Fig. 12-2). But these have to be handled in a precise manner when dealing with the argon laser. This is what we do: We usually use small 50-μ spot-size coagulations with multiple pulsed impacts; this is usually a place for a sweeping movement or a painting movement with the argon laser, simply because one might run into other vital structures such as the large arteries or veins in the background. Also, as was well demonstrated by Dr. Goldberg, you have to recognize vessels that are intimately approximated to the surface of the disc because the vessels will absorb the heat, as will patches of hemorrhage or pigment; and converting this light into heat would then cause a disruption of the nerve fiber layer. But with pulsed impacts, perhaps of 0.05 or 0.1 of a second, this neovascularization can be obliterated. This is the pre-op appearance of an epipapillary area of neovascularization (Fig. 12-3). The end point for this type of photocoagulation technique is a morphologic change, not a coagulation; that is, once the vessel has entered the vitreous it is rather rare that you will see a graying or white coagulation that you see back in the pigment epithelium. You actually see a morphologic change.

Again, the effect that one wishes to create, after sorting out the feeder vessel, is to put the feeder vessel into spasm in order to sequester and to capture the blood in the frond. One then paints back and forth over the more distal frond with a

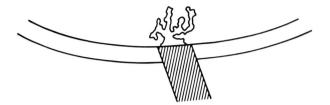

Fig. 12-1. Diagram of typical epipapillary neovascularization.

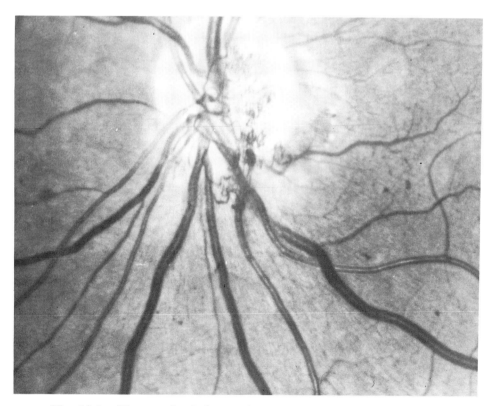

Fig. 12-2. Photograph of characteristic epipapillary neovascularization.

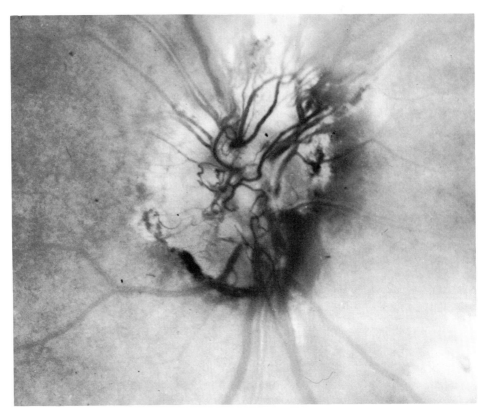

Fig. 12-3. Epipapillary neovascularization prior to argon laser photocoagulation (cf. Figs. 12-4 and 12-5).

larger size beam—perhaps 100 to 150 μ—with a slightly higher power than used with the 50-μ beam, in order to coagulate the blood that is now remaining in the vessels themselves. The vessels in Figure 12-4 have been segmented and have been thrown into spasm; the frond itself has been treated with larger coagulations. Approximately 6 to 8 weeks later the glial scar remains with no evidence of neovascularization (Fig. 12-5). Cases such as this will do extremely well for long periods of time.

The next type is the peripapillary neovascularization (Fig. 12-6). This is the type that extends a short distance over the retina in a radial type of distribution. It usually has a circumferential vessel, and the supply, the feeder, and the collector vessels are located just inside the rim of the optic nerve. Here, again, the point is to find the feeder by fluorescein angiography or by direct inspection, and then to coagulate at the feeder area; many times one does not have to go too far off the disc rim. However, in the more difficult types the technique is to coagulate on the disc rim and then to go radially from the optic disc, causing as little damage as possible. Of course photocoagulation in the papillomacular bundle zone should be minimal. And this has caused obliteration in a rather high percentage of cases, somewhere approximating 60-percent obliteration over a 6-month period, which we have taken as the time for what we call "true obliteration." That is, other areas of neovascularization may grow from an old treated area, but once we have treated

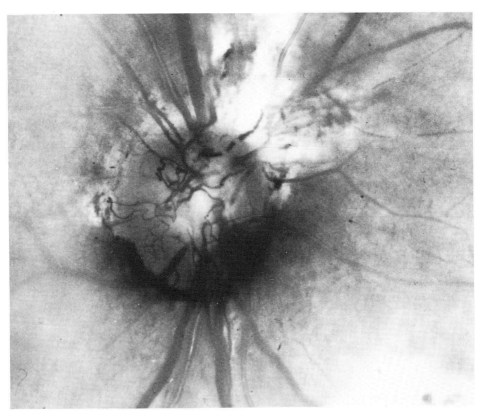

Fig. 12-4. Epipapillary neovascularization immediately after argon laser photocoagulation (cf. Figs. 12-3 and 12-5).

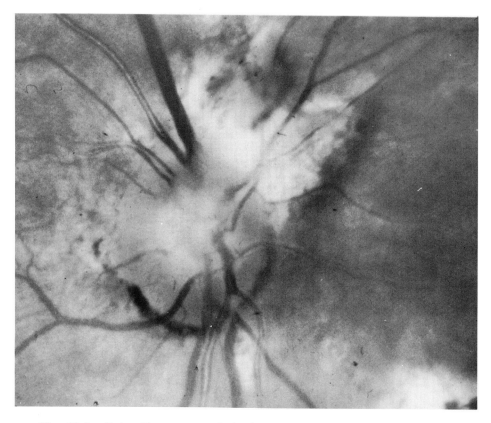

Fig. 12-5. Epipapillary neovascularization 2 months after argon laser photocoagulation (cf. Figs. 12-3 and 12-4).

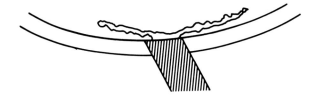

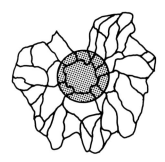

Fig. 12-6.   Diagram of typical peripapillary neovascularization.

this area it has to remain obliterated for 6 months in order for us to consider it a success.

Figure 12-7 shows an early type of neovascularization of the peripapillary type; the tufts are forming at the disc and are moving peripherally. If you wait 3 or 4 weeks, it will be out beyond the macula; if you wait another month or two, it will be out to the distal arcades. It is one of the less difficult to treat. The easiest to treat, of course, is surface neovascularization—which we will discuss—because we have the help of the pigment epithelium to obliterate it. We can obliterate most of these vessels and they will remain this way for long periods of time.

Usually peripapillary neovascularization grows very shallowly over perhaps the posterior hyaloid attachment to the disc. It does not seem to grow on the internal limiting membrane; it extends little into the vitreous, more like a very shallow saucer. Just a short period of about 3 weeks later we have obliterated the frond. As it turned out, this went on and did extremely well without any proliferation except for a small area about 5 or 6 months later.

A 21-year-old girl had a huge and well-entrenched shunting system, hemorrhages, and bizarre neovascularization all over the retina. Treating in the same way, segmentation of the shunts by photocoagulation was accomplished with a rather high intensity; in those days, we could use a 40-μ spot size because we were using an open-ended system. She is completely dry and has 20/20 vision 4.5 years later;

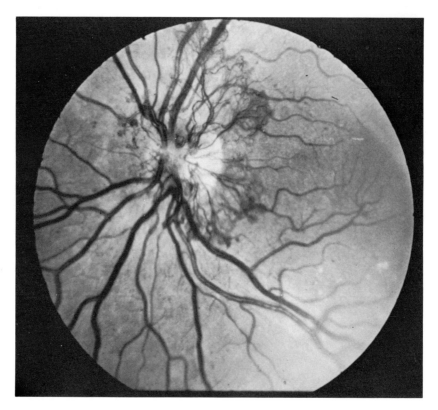

Fig. 12-7. Photograph of characteristic peripapillary neovascularization.

a scotoma can be demonstrated which corresponds to the area of photocoagulation, but no sector defect.

Figure 12-8 shows another case with a tremendous amount of peripapillary neovascularization with hemorrhages at the distal portion of the circumferential ring. Figure 12-9 shows what the patient looked like immediately after treatment. We had coagulated much of the neovascularization, but the main channels were still well formed and, of course, the neovascular proliferation stimulus could activate any one of these at any time. We went ahead and retreated again, trying to stay away from the macular zone if we could. Finally, after several other treatments, she still has 20/25 vision and has no sign of any neovascularization (Fig. 12-10).

Now, as we come to the next types of neovascularization, we are getting a bit away from the pigment epithelium and moving into the vitreous. These types are either the retinovitreal type or the papillovitreal type. The retinovitreal type usually grows along an old hemorrhage where the fibrin has been formed from a spray of blood into the vitreous. The neovascularization extends up along the fibrin like a trellis work. The neovascularization can also form upon itself and surround itself with glial tissue; it then grows a bit farther and fortifies itself with glial proliferation, and this can extend a great distance into the vitreous.

And, of course, the last type that we see most commonly is coming up along the back surface of the posterior hyaloid. The idea is to treat this and to obliterate these zones, by the feeder vessel spasm, and treating the frond itself once the

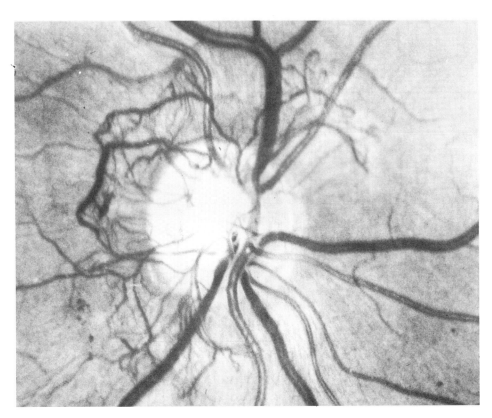

Fig. 12-8. Peripapillary neovascularization prior to argon laser photocoagulation (cf. Figs. 12-9 and 12-10).

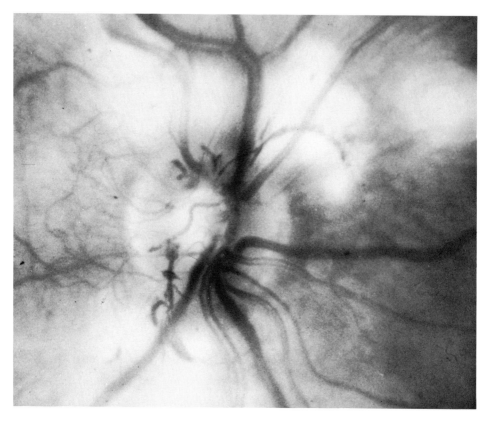

Fig. 12-9. Peripapillary neovascularization immediately after argon laser photo-coagulation (cf. Figs. 12-8 and 12-10).

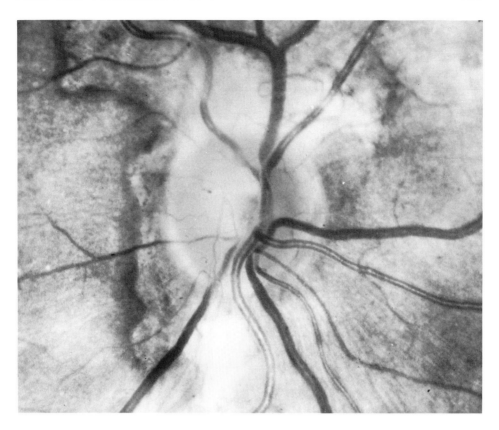

Fig. 12-10.   Peripapillary neovascularization 6 weeks after argon laser photocoagulation (cf. Figs. 12-8 and 12-9).

blood has been sequestered. And one has to do this coagulation with a very small amount of energy. I think this is where the argon laser is most important, among other things, since it just cannot be done with any other photocoagulation system. You have to put in an extremely small amount of energy and stay away from the infrared part of the spectrum because this is the spectral zone that will cause posterior hyaloid shrinkage. I am sure it is the thing that contributes to the degree of macular pucker that has been reported in xenon arc cases.

The papillovitreal neovascularization extends along the posterior hyaloid. This is the type that I call the arcuate type of papillovitreal neovascularization; it simply looks like an arc (Fig. 12-11). It corresponds to the distribution that Dr. Goldberg talked about (Chapter 8) which is supratemporal and the most common. The infratemporal involvement is the next most common, then supranasal and infranasal. Another type—a columnar type—is very easy to treat because there are usually only one or two feeders and maybe three collector vessels. There is also a confluent papillovitreal type which is extremely difficult to treat because there are many feeder vessels (Fig. 12-12). In the confluent types that Hunter Little demonstrated in Chapter 11, you must do a precise job in locating the feeder vessel with fluorescein angiography.

Two stages of fronds exist for each of the arcuate, columnar, and confluent types;

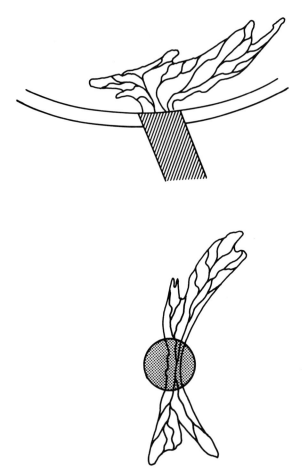

Fig. 12-11. Diagram of typical papillovitreal neovascularization.

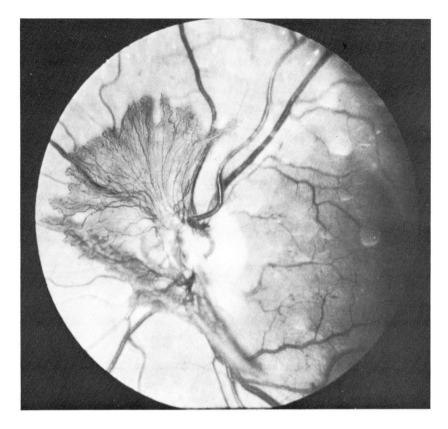

Fig. 12-12.   Photograph of characteristic papillovitreal neovascularization.

these are the immature and mature stages. The immature has a large amount of vascularity; it has not yet reinforced itself, as it does in old age, with a lot of glial proliferation. The therapeutic technique in these is to coagulate the feeder and then to irradiate the frond, and obliterate and coagulate as much as you can up along the frond itself. The technique, however, differs from the mature type of papillovitreal frond; these are usually well entrenched and well fortified with glial proliferation down along the stalk. The vessels are large, and if you try to partially coagulate them with the laser, you will find that you usually end up causing a large hemorrhage. However, the place where you find the greatest danger, and which should be checked at each office visit, is along the border of the mature papillo-vitreal frond where endothelial budding may be occurring. The endothelial buds cannot stand even a slight rise in pressure. They are very fragile and they break; and, as you have all seen, there are rivulets of blood coming from them frequently. I usually look at these with either the slit lamp or by direct ophthalmoscopy; if I see these little areas, I will treat them as indicated. This is all I will treat in the mature papillovitreal frond.

This is an immature, very fleshy papillovitreal frond (Fig. 12-13). Figure 12-14 shows the eye right after treatment. About 7 weeks later there is complete obliteration (Fig. 12-15). As you can see, the patient had other problems that were also taken care of. It is interesting to note that after treatment, if the frond

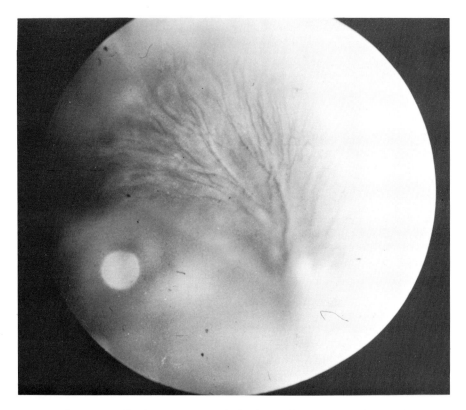

Fig. 12-13. Papillovitreal neovascularization prior to argon laser photocoagulation (cf. Figs. 12-14 and 12-15).

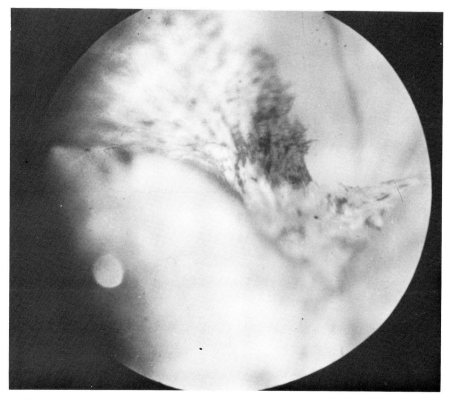

Fig. 12-14.   Papillovitreal neovascularization immediately after argon laser photocoagulation (cf. Figs. 12-13 and 12-15).

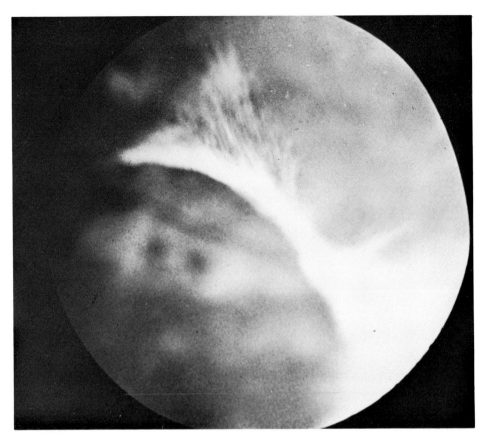

Fig. 12-15. Papillovitreal neovascularization 7 weeks after argon laser photocoagulation (cf. Figs. 12-13 and 12-14).

proliferates or if a new area of neovascularization develops, it many times will be of the immature type. It will grow rapidly and be extremely vascular, with very little fortification by glial tissue. With long columnar types we create a spasm and then treat around the distal frond. The krypton laser has no real advantage at the present time over the argon laser. But by coagulating the feeder and the distal neovascularization, an excellent job can be done in this type of papillovitreal neovascularization. As Dr. Little pointed out in Chapter 11, any type of argon laser photocoagulation of retinovitreal neovascularization is a never-ending job. We are not reducing the stimulus, whatever it is, to this type of proliferation, but we can go ahead and do our best to try to reinforce it or obliterate it. Many times, because they are sequestered with these bigger, more mature types of fronds, you will run into the difficulty that I have experienced frequently, that is, it is hard to find the feeders and you have to perform some coagulations of extremely high power on the area that you think is the feeder area. Many times you may not get that vessel completely occluded; and if you do not, the distal vessels are less easy to obliterate. In one case we did obliterate most feeder vessels but one of the feeder vessels was open, and so we had what really amounted to partial venous occlusion. However, it was enough, as is usually the case, to convert it into an avascular glial strand 3 to 4 months later; the strand has remained unchanged for nearly 4 years.

The retinovitreal type of neovascularization (Fig. 12-16) is much like the papillovitreal, but is coming from the vitreal vessels rather than the disc. It is growing up along a footplate from a highly detached posterior hyaloid that is inserted in the retina (Fig. 12-17).

Figure 12-18 shows an area with retinovitreal neovascularization and well entrenched vessels, with its blood supply from a major vein (Fig. 12-18). The idea here is to attack this region in order to obliterate the entire area, which has been difficult in many cases of this type. But if you go after it as well as you can and try to leave the main vein draining behind it, you end up with the main channels, but no areas of growth (Fig. 12-19). If you follow this along with fluorescein you will find that there is no growth (Fig. 12-20). This patient has remained about a year without new growth at all in any areas.

One woman had a huge frond coming up into the vitreous, in her only eye, that was bleeding at about 4- to 5-week intervals. She would clear up and then go down to 20/60 or 20/70 because of the vitreous bleed. Obviously, because of the vitreous traction in the large frond, it would be impossible to treat this whole area.

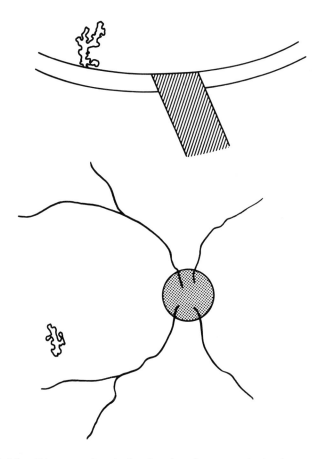

Fig. 12-16. Diagram of typical retinovitreal neovascularization.

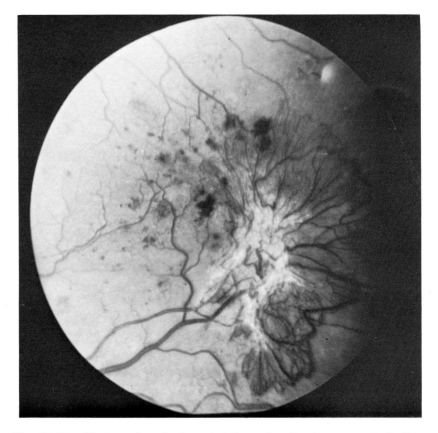

Fig. 12-17. Photograph of characteristic retinovitreal neovascularization.

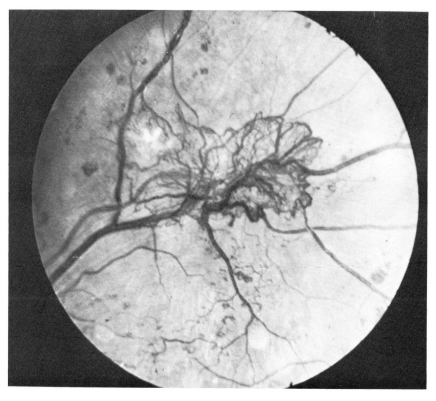

Fig. 12-18. Retinovitreal neovascularization prior to argon laser photocoagulation (cf. Figs. 12-19 and 12-20).

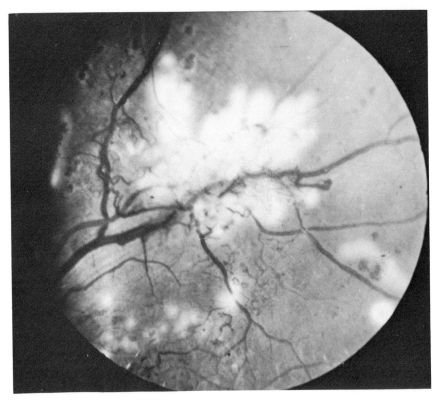

Fig. 12-19. Retinovitreal neovascularization immediately after argon laser photo-coagulation (cf. Figs. 12-18 and 12-20).

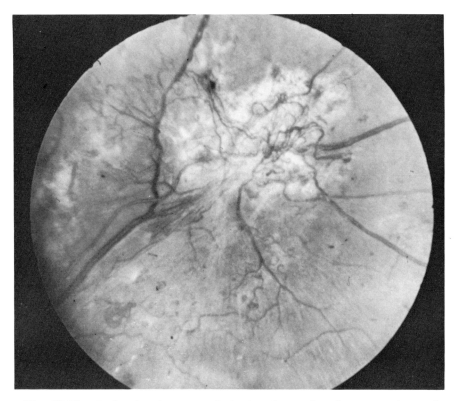

Fig. 12-20. Retinovitreal neovascularization 2 months after argon laser photocoagulation (cf. Figs. 12-18 and 12-19).

Echoing some of the remarks of Dr. Goldberg, the arterioles are extremely difficult to photocoagulate. In fact, if you just treat the arteriole directly, it is almost impossible with the argon or any source to obliterate an arteriole due to its high flow system. The way to coagulate an arteriole is to throw an area into spasm, and to throw it into spasm a short distance distally. Then you sweep over the intervening area of vessel with a very light, relatively low power. In effect, you have a kind of entrapment of blood and you are slowly coagulating that region. You do not want to rupture it, of course, but you can coagulate without much difficulty. About 3 or 4 weeks later the whole arteriole was segmented. After about a year the patient has had no repeated hemorrhages. This is one of the techniques that you sometimes must employ for the more severe retinovitreal types of neovascularization.

The last type is the preretinal, or surface type neovascularization which again extends along the surface of the internal limiting membrane (Fig. 12-21). These are easier to obliterate because they are nearer to the pigment epithelium.

In a similar example of surface neovascularization, there are a few vessels coming back to the disc for neovascularization, so we might even call this a combination of peripapillary and surface neovascularization (Fig. 12-22).

The young girl in Figure 12-23 had 20/20 vision. We treated her with 50-μ spots at about 200 or 250 mW (Fig. 12-23). It is at these power densities that the complications arise. In the last year we have had about 3 percent complications and most all have been from small areas of neovascularization and patches

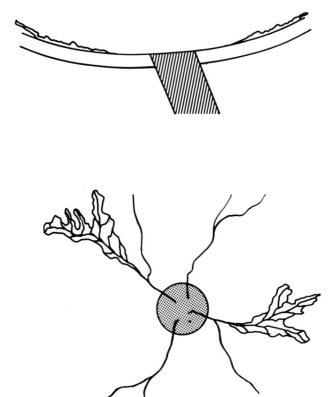

Fig. 12-21. Diagram of typical preretinal neovascularization.

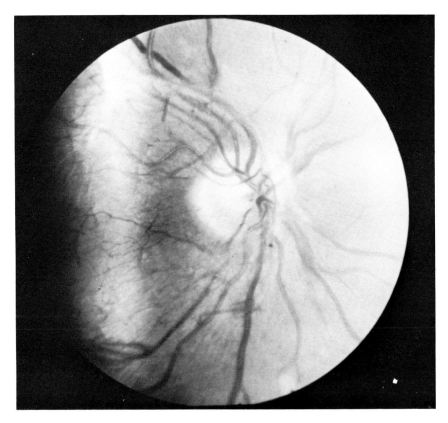

Fig. 12-22. Photograph of preretinal neovascularization prior to argon laser photocoagulation (cf. Figs. 12-23 and 12-24).

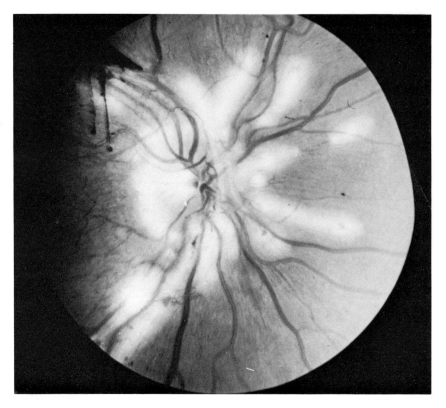

Fig. 12-23. Preretinal neovascularization immediately after argon laser photocoagulation (cf. Figs. 12-22 and 12-24).

of glial proliferation. They dry up in about 10 days to 2 weeks, or perhaps a
week longer. They have not caused any trouble, but they do occur, and this is
one of the small hazards; but you have to treat them heavily in order to get the
result of obliteration of the neovascularization. The patient has gone about 2.5
years without regrowth of neovascularization. She has some macular strias, but
this still does not prevent her from retaining the 20/20 vision that she had prior
to photocoagulation (Fig. 12-24).

In another eye, again with 20/20 vision, there were big footplates coming
down into the paramacular area and some glial proliferation. This girl still has
20/20 vision; field defect corresponds to the coagulated area but there has been
no regrowth of neovascularization for about a 3-year period.

I would like to outline our examination routine for the diabetic patients. We
examine the potential diabetic every 2 years. I think this is a good system. We
examine the overt diabetic, from the onset of diabetes, every year with Kodachrome
fundus photography. Once they start getting into any difficulty ophthalmoscopically,
we convert to a 6-months' examination interval when we do Kodachrome fundus
photography and fluorescein angiography. This documents the microangiopathy,
which is usually much worse than we can see ophthalmoscopically. Once we
get into the area of the late nonproliferative or the early proliferative diabetic
retinopathy, the xenon arc, as Dr. Okun so nicely pointed out, the ruby laser,

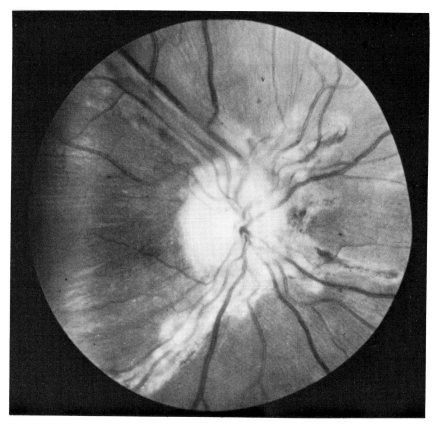

Fig. 12-24. Preretinal neovascularization 6 weeks after argon laser photocoagulation (cf. Figs. 12-22 and 12-23).

that Dr. Aiello has worked out so well in Boston, and the argon laser, all have great use. Once you get into the late proliferative phase with the disc and the intravitreal neovascularization, the only instrument in my experience that works with any degree of success, is the argon laser. Of course, once we get into the stage of retinal detachment the whole subject of retinal surgery must be explored. So I hope that, if you have not tried the argon laser, or any of these photocoagulation techniques, you will consider their great promise. I think that these devices expand our therapeutic armamentarium and, coupled to greater diagnostic capabilities, will lead us to a more constructive rationale for the treatment of all phases of diabetic retinopathy.

Chapter 13
Panel Discussions

Dr. Snyder. The preceding four speakers have done an excellent job of covering some of the pros and cons of the various entities here. There is one that deserves some mention before we get into the written questions. Dr. Okun, I would appreciate brief comments from you on the handling of diabetic retinal detachment.

Dr. Okun. In spite of everything that we do for the diabetic patient in attempting to save him from this fate, some patients nevertheless will go on to a traction type of retinal detachment. Very expert ophthalmoscopic examinations are required to differentiate the fibrovascular membranes from the retina, and the retinoschisis from the detachment, particularly if the vitreous has been partially opacified by repeated hemorrhages. If you can master an examination of this type of eye, you have mastered indirect ophthalmoscopy.

If any retinal breaks are found, they must be closed. Unfortunately, the retinal breaks in eyes with proliferative diabetic retinopathy are located extremely posteriorly, usually in close association with fibrous membranes. Closure of these breaks is usually difficult as is the drainage of subretinal fluid. But breaks as close as one disc diameter from the disc can be closed, particularly if subretinal fluid is successfully evacuated. Now, if there are no breaks, and it is strictly a traction type of retinal detachment, I feel that some type of scleral buckling procedure should be performed.* By indenting each quadrant of the preequatorial sclera with a cotton stick applicator, one can determine in which quadrant a buckling procedure would produce the greatest relaxation of the traction. If there is no difference, then an encircling procedure is performed, with drainage of subretinal fluid whenever possible, The essential therapeutic factors are (1) to buckle the retina at the site of greatest traction, and (2) to drain subretinal fluid whenever possible. By deforming the globe, the intravitreal volume is reduced and, provided there is no loss of formed vitreous, this loss is accomplished by absorption or evacuation of liquid subretinal fluid or liquified vitreous.

We have been doing buckling procedures on diabetics for approximately 15

---

* Okun E, Johnston GP, Boniuk I: Management of Diabetic Retinopathy; A Stereoscopic Presentation. St. Louis, Mosby, 1971, pp 142–154.

Table 13-1

Diabetic Retinal Detachment—Surgical Procedures

Type of Buckling	No. eyes	No. Eyes With Useful Vision (%)	No. Eyes with 20/400 or Better (%)	Average Length Follow-up (months)
Encircling with resection	38	24 (63)	19 (50)	38
Encircling without resection but with plombage	14	8 (57)	5 (36)	17
Episcleral encircling	25	19 (76)	14 (56)	18
Resection alone	3	3 (100)	3 (100)	67
Primary liquid silicone	1	0 (0)	0 (0)	6
Total	81	54 (67)	41 (51)	29

years now, and this experience has taught us that the operation is definitely of
value, providing there is some potential function remaining in the eye. A particularly good candidate is a patient who has been followed with good macular function,
who suddenly loses that function secondary to retinal detachment. On the other
hand, one who comes to you for the first time with a large membrane that obscures
most of the posterior pole will not benefit from detachment surgery. The retina
which is very slightly detached, due entirely to tangential traction, is extremely
difficult to improve with any type of surgery. In my experience these cases don't
do nearly as well as the detachments that have more fluid. Table 13-1 shows the
results of various types of buckling procedures that we have performed for diabetic
detachments. The overall success rate in terms of visual improvement is 67 percent.
In terms of eyes which retain 20/400 or better visual acuity, which is really
something for these people, the success rate is 51 percent. It did not seem to
make any difference whether or not retinal breaks were present (Table 13-2).
Success in retinal detachment surgery on these eyes cannot be measured in terms
of getting the entire retina completely flat, because it usually is not possible to
flatten the retina at the point where the traction is highest. What we should aim
for is flattening as much of the retina as will go back.

Table 13-3 attempts to shed some light on the question of whether or not
subretinal fluid should be drained. However, these data are somewhat biased in
terms of no drainage of subretinal fluid because they include a series of cases that
were buckled before the macula was involved. In contrast to the usual rhegmatogenous detachment in which the first area to settle back is the macula, in these
diabetic traction detachments the macula is the last area to settle back because

Table 13-2

Diabetic Retinal Detachment—Presence or Absence of Holes

Preoperative Condition	No. Eyes	With Useful Vision (%)	With 20/400 or Better (%)
Detachment without breaks	47	31 (66)	23 (49)
Detachment with breaks	34	22 (65)	18 (53)

Table 13–3

Drainage of SRF

	No. Eyes	With Useful Vision (%)	With 20/400 or Better (%)
SRF	59	38 (64)	28 (47)
No SRF	22	16 (73)	13 (59)

that's where most of the traction is. So when the macula is detached, I personally like to drain subretinal fluid.

Dr. Vaiser. Francis, have you found that laser treatment over the nerve head has produced clinically observable fiber bundle defects?

Dr. L'Esperance. I do not remember our slide specifically. When we first started we were using 40-μ spots and even 35-μ spots. We were going down to the smallest focus that the eye was capable of producing. And using rather high energies, as with anything else, we did not know what the end result should be. Therefore, using higher power densities, smaller impact diameters, and higher inputs, I did get some sector defects. I think, as I recall, it was about 0.4 to 0.5 percent of the cases that we treated in 1968. Since that time, observing strictly the rules of not treating in areas of hemorrhage on the disc, of any pigment on the disc, and staying away from any vessels that seem to be large and that could conceivably produce a great deal of heat on the disc itself, we have not had any sector defects. Diabetics, as you know, are very difficult to measure by perimetry, simply because, as was stated this morning, many of them have field defects to begin with and most of them perhaps have a rather dull retina anyway; and with this dull retina, they go without field loss symptoms. I'm sure in my own mind that several of our cases have had field defects which could not be picked up on the perimeter.

Dr. Vaiser. How do you feel about the use of the argon laser versus the xenon?

Dr. L'Esperance. I'd just like to throw some support to what Dr. Okun presented (Chapter 10). I use the xenon in about 25 to 30 percent of the cases, and I use it for several reasons. First, the West German Zeiss provides a great deal of magnification—about 15 magnifications. Looking through the handle and with the bright light is extremely advantageous because you can see some areas of neovascularization that you cannot see even by prior examination in the office. Second, the thing that I alluded to somewhat during my presentation was the fact that the xenon arc does have the infrared components. It has all the wavelengths from 4000 to 16,000 Å, and this infrared must not be considered lightly, because it does two things; it perhaps causes a bit more complications, but it does have some facets that are advantageous, that is, it has greater penetration and, in some of the earlier cases of diabetic retinopathy, perhaps when you have some surface glial proliferation, you have neovascularization mixed in with it. Or you may have a large mass of vascular tissue, large tortuous vessels that are neovascular. These, to be treated with the argon, cause a surface effect on the hemoglobin bolus and certainly with glial proliferation there is a change. Argon light would be scattered by the glial tissue and therefore you would either use higher energy or not get an adequate result for these reasons. Therefore, with very early proliferative diabetic retinopathy, or late nonproliferative diabetic retinopathy, I will use the zenon arc.

Another thing which should be kept in mind is the fact that with all the wavelengths of the xenon output, there are those which the retinal structures absorb a little differently. For some reason the nerve fiber layer will pick up at one wavelength and not at another. All of the nuclear elements will have high absorption complexes. All of these structures in the retina will absorb parts of this huge presentation of wavelengths that the xenon arc has; and, therefore, what you can get is a shriveling of the retina around, let's say, intraretinal vessels, or even on surface vessels that sometimes is difficult to accomplish with the argon. The argon, remember, is absorbed almost completely unless you go to higher powers, as was demonstrated in Dr. Goldberg's paper (Chapter 8); but usually at the lower powers it is absorbed almost completely by pigment such as melanin or hemoglobin. And therefore you have to expect the heat to be generated, reflected back from the pigment epithelium or, if the vessel is small enough, to constrict and coagulate the vessel or, perhaps if it's a large vessel, just to have a surface effect. All of these things have to be weighed. I'd like to leave the impression that the argon laser does things that no other photocoagulation system can do. It can be used in the place of the xenon photocoagulator in many many conditions, but there are some that I think should be thought about more, and I wholeheartedly second what Dr. Okun stated earlier.

Dr. Vaiser. Would Dr. Zweng have any comments to make regarding the different types of photocoagulation systems?

Dr. Zweng. If one wishes to get a greater radiation from the retinal pigment epithelium (RPE) area, both into the choroid and up into the intraretinal layers, he should use a larger spot size than 50 or 100 μ. This is true for the following reason: This is a three-dimensional lesion; the central part does not have a nonheated area to radiate out into and cool; therefore it stays hotter longer in the larger spot sizes than the smaller. By larger we mean 500 to 1000 μ, with the 200-μ spot size being intermediate and the 100-μ and the 50-μ being small. A longer time exposure gives the same effect. One can get, therefore, a lesion that is thicker by using the larger spot size and a longer exposure time with argon laser photocoagulation.

All this discussion comparing one photocoagulation system with the other makes me want to show the two figures. All photocoagulation systems are composed of three elements: the light source (argon or ruby laser or xenon arc); the delivery system—the way in which that light is delivered onto the retina—direct, modified, indirect ophthalmoscope or the slit lamp; and the operator. Of the elements, the operator is by far the most variable depending upon his training, his experience, and his interest. A group of ophthalmologists have given a good deal of their time and professional energy to the field of photocoagulation in diabetic retinopathy; and the results that any one of us gets may or not be duplicated by others depending upon training, experience, and interest. Some can do very clever things with the direct-viewing xenon arc photocoagulator that many others cannot duplicate. Others can be very expert with argon laser slit-lamp photocoagulation. So, as these discussions progress, I suggest that you keep that factor in mind and read the literature. Above all, if you are interested in doing photocoagulation in diabetic retinopathy, do acquire training, develop experience, and maintain interest, or you simply won't do as good a job as can be done.

Dr. Vaiser. Dr. Hutton, why wouldn't thickening of the basement membrane in capillaries alone account for microaneurysm formation?

Dr. Hutton. The available literature, primarily the light microscopic studies of Cogan and Kuwabara * and the electron microscopic studies of Toussaint and Duistin,† though they define basement membrane thickening, couldn't really correlate this directly with the development of microaneurysms. So, although it's a nice approach, so far it just cannot be reproduced on histologic studies.

Dr. Vaiser. Dr. Kohner, is it possible that the vascular reaction to the fluorescein itself could account for the daily fluctuation of values you have seen in your studies?

Dr. Kohner: I did not take fluorescein angiograms on consecutive days, although in a few patients I have done it twice within the same sitting, that is, within 10 minutes. The nearest thing between two consecutive transit time estimations was 6 weeks. I do not think that fluorescein would cause any vascular reaction of the sort you envisage. Fluorescein, on the whole, is not a toxic substance, although about a year ago there was a paper in the American Journal of Ophthalmology which stated that fluorescein causes vascular dilatation. I do not think this is so. The reason why vessels look wider on fluorescein angiograms than on color photographs is due to the fact that on color photographs you only see the red cell column and miss the plasma zone, which is clearly shown on fluorescein angiograms.

Dr. Vaiser. Dr. Siperstein, would you discuss the ability to detect basement membrane thickening in quadriceps muscle capillary prior to the onset of the carbohydrate abnormalities of diabetes? Have others found data which agree or disagree with your findings? How does the duration of overt hyperglycemia affect basement membrane thickening?

Dr. Siperstein. There has been some disagreement at various meetings regarding these points. Our group has shown that as many as 83 percent of prediabetics will show basement membrane thickening before their carbohydrate intolerance occurs. Candrini and Bloodworth have now confirmed this finding.

We find that there is thickening of basement membrane in the majority of patients at the time of onset of the earliest evidence of significant glucose abnormalities; there is no further thickening for at least 10 to 20 years. Though his discussion of these points is a little obscure and his method yields a lower incidence of basement membrane thickening than does ours, Williamson has confirmed both of these findings in the August 1972 issue of *Diabetes*.

Dr. Vaiser. Marvin, what, if any, is the relationship between thickening of the basement membrane and capillary nonfilling?

---

* Cogan D, Kuwabara T: Vascular Complications of Diabetes Mellitus. St. Louis, Mosby, 1967, p 55

† Toussaint D, Duistin P: Electron Microscopy of Normal and Diabetic Retinal Capillaries, Arch Ophthal 70:140, 1963

Dr. Siperstein. I cannot answer the question since I do not know, and I am not familiar with the phenomenon. If you are indicating that capillaries in muscle in the diabetic do not fill, I'm not aware of that.

Dr. Vaiser. I was hoping you would generalize beyond the muscle if possible. Certainly basement membrane thickening is a universal phenomenon. I am not personally familiar with the capillary bed in the muscle, but elsewhere in the body there is certainly widespread occlusion and nonfilling of the capillaries. So the question really tries to bring together two essentially universal and almost omnipresent phenomena in the microvasculature of the diabetic; is there any known relationship between basement membrane thickening and nonfilling of the capillary bed?

Dr. Siperstein. I do not know. You'll find me very careful when it comes to putting together the anatomic findings and any physiologic implications of those findings. The only tissue about which I feel at all confident in making this association is in the kidney. And here the capillary and the glomerulus is destroyed by thickening of the basement membrane. The kidney literally is replaced by masses of basement membrane. Then there is no question that capillary filling is impaired. Beyond that I think we are almost totally ignorant as to the physiologic or the detailed pathologic implications of thickening of the basement membrane in any other tissues.

Dr. Vaiser. Dr. Caird, had all the patients in your study been followed from time of diagnosis? How does the panel feel about early good diabetic control versus later good control and the incidence of malignant retinopathy? Any statistics?

Dr. Snyder. By malignant, do you mean PDR?

Dr. Vaiser. The way Dr. Caird mentioned it, yes.

Dr. Caird. The data I showed (Chapter 5) came from two sources. One was a large collection of some 2000 patients, not all of whom had been followed from the time diabetes was first diagnosed. The restricted collection of 300 patients, where I discussed the relationship between control and development of retinopathy, had all been followed from the time of diagnosis for the 10 to 15 years necessary for them to enter the investigation.

Dr. Vaiser. Hunter, in how many sessions do you accomplish the 360-degree peripheral retinal ablation?

Dr. Little. As I stated, these should include about 600 to 1200 lesions, usually in the neighborhood of 1000 lesions, in addition to those applied to the disc. I have done this in one session, but I do not recommend it. I recommend that they be done in two or three sessions. What I usually do is have the patient with all his information—studies and magnifications—all set and we heat up the laser, focusing on the feeder vessels and the frond at the disc. At that sitting I'll go perhaps 180 degrees above. Then I bring the patient back the next day, and probably repeat the fluorescein to see if the vessels on the disc are reopened; and if it is obvious that they have reopened, there is no need to do the fluorescein. But the second day after the initial treatment, the patient is re-treated, again to the frond on the disc, to make certain that you have obliterated the feeder and the entire frond, and then complete the ablation. So there are usually two sessions. I think I mentioned that in one case, where there was extensive proliferans off the disc, so-called nude vessels, there was very little connective tissue element. It was just a perfect one to get movies on. I treated 360 degrees in the periphery first because our photographer was not there that day and I wanted him to be there to get pictures of the feeder vessel/frond treatment. So I brought the patient back in 4 or 5 days to do this; in the meantime she bled. What I think had happened is that with the extensive ablation (and I do not mean just a few lesions, but 1000 such lesions applied just everywhere I could put them), you obliterate many many capillaries, and in such a case I am certain that we have altered the hemodynamics. The patient had increased pressure, most likely at the disc vessel, because she had a sizable hemorrhage resulting therefrom. What I am recommending is that if you do ablation only, as Dr. Zweng is doing now, I think the best approach would be to do it stepwise, so that you really don't shock the retina with any sudden change in hemodynamics. You might break it into three sessions, at least. If you are going to first treat the vessels on the disc, so you essentially knock that out, then I think you can probably get away with doing a bit more ablation.

Dr. Vaiser. Why haven't you used the xenon arc photocoagulator for the past 3 years? Is the instrument that bad?

Dr. Little. Why not xenon? I don't object to the xenon. It's just that I find that the argon in my hands is easier to operate, the spot size used for ablation around the major arcade diopter to the midperiphery is a 500-μ spot, 0.5 mm; and then for the far periphery we can use the 1000-μ spot, which is about the size you would be using if you use the xenon. I enjoy sitting down when I do it rather than bending over. I always got a back pain when I used the xenon; but I think that as far as ablation is concerned, either instrument is satisfactory. Then you can bring out all the other theoretical differences. I don't know whether they are important or not. Increased infrared heat and all that sort of thing. I don't know whether it's good or bad—I really don't think it makes any difference which instrument you use. My feeling is that if you are going to have the patient seated there and you are going to treat a feeder and frond with the argon, why should you pick him up and go across the room or go across town to use the xenon. I have not found this necessary. The only time I use the xenon now is in Coats' disease, when I have to put the patient to sleep, which I did a year ago. And I treated a malignant melanoma and used the xenon for that. But those are the only 2 cases I have used xenon on in the last 2 years.

Dr. Vaiser. May I say one thing in relation to that? I personally have had several cases that have had reduced vision following ablation and I feel that in my cases this was due to macular edema.

Dr. Kohner. Our group has used xenon arc for peripheral photocoagulation of large retinal areas in the treatment of diabetic retinopathy. In some such patients there was decrease in vision not due to macular edema. This work will be reported by Dr. Boulton shortly.

Dr. Snyder. Any comments, Dr. Zweng?

Dr. Zweng. May we have the third and fourth slides that I gave? These show a drawing and table of the size lesions that we use, and how Dr. Little and I are doing this 360-degree so-called ablation which we now call pan-retinal photo-coagulation (PRP). In the macular area we use a 50- to 100-μ spot size at 0.1 seconds, 100 to 200 mW down. In addition to PRP, we treat leaking areas in the paramacular area; the spot size is a little larger—100 to 200 μ at 0.2 seconds, from 0.1 to 0.2 seconds, and then 100 to 300 mW. Now these are guidelines, and as one accumulates experience, as always with guidelines, one can deviate from them. But these are good things to start with; and then along the major vessels, inside the major vessels, the superior and inferior vascular arcade size, we use 200- and 500-μ spot size, 0.1 to 0.2 seconds, and 200 to 500 mW. Then beyond the major vessels 500 to 1000 μ at 0.1 to 0.2 seconds and 500 to 1500 mW. Many of you might question 1500 mW. Well, the Coherent Radiation Laboratory's instrument can deliver into the eye almost 2000 mW, but the dial which is furnished with the instrument now will only go up to 1000 mW. But we found that when you are up to 1000 μ, if you want to stay at 0.1 seconds you usually have to go over 1000 mW; so, knowing that it had a greater output, we asked for a dial that will go up higher than 1000 mW. It is now available and I think that those of you who have the instrument should write Coherent Radiation and ask them for whatever charge they make to retrofit, to have that capability available, because the energy and the power are in the machine. Next slide shows this in a little drawing that gives hopefully the same information, though a bit more graphically. And you have to go right out to the equator; as far as I personally am concerned, we have not done what we want to do with this unless we can document some optic atrophy. I think that is essential if one has any chance at all to rid the nerve head of the neovascularization. I think the induction of some optic atrophy is essential. Sometimes, perhaps, you have to go beyond the equator. I also think the posterior pole is an area of higher metabolic activity than the far periphery, so treating focal pathology in the macula and in the macular papillary bundle, I think is also an important component in this cutting down on the amount of retina needing to be oxygenated.

Dr. Vaiser. Dr. Davis, do we have any statistics regarding the percentage of recurrence after a spontaneous remission has occurred?

Dr. Davis. I can't really give you any good numbers. I hope that a year from now I can give you good numbers about the patients we have followed for many years now. In general, I would say the percentage is not very high. The patient that I presented (Chapter 2), who regressed again, is unusual. I think most patients who look burned out but still have useful vision usually do pretty well. They may have a small vitreous hemorrhage a year later that clears; I really cannot give you good data, I can only give you my clinical impression.

Dr. Vaiser. The engorged appearance of some cases of diabetic retinopathy is similar to that seen in venous occlusion. What is the basis for this?

Dr. Davis. Well, we could talk for a long time on that. This appearance has been used—it appears in the literature in a sort of conjectural way to suggest there must be some sort of venous obstruction in diabetic retinopathy. But some of the experimental work, I believe of Dr. S. S. Hayreh, shows that in monkeys one has to partially occlude the arterial as well as the venous circulation to get a typical vein occlusion. That work, I think, fits with my preconception of diabetic retinopathy;

there is partial occlusion upstream, partial obliteration of the capillary bed, and there ought to be a reasonable cause for venous dilatation downstream. I have thought about it in a rather simplistic way, thinking that the veins are dilated because they are ischemic too, because there is not enough blood getting through the arterioles and capillaries into the veins, and the veins are dilated—not because there is obstruction downstream towards the disc, but because of obstruction upstream in the capillary bed. If one accepts that reasoning, then it is not surprising that the veins are dilated in the diabetic. If you do not accept that reasoning, then I am perplexed and I cannot give you any other answer. I don't really think there is an element of venous obstruction in the central retinal vein in diabetic retinopathy.

Dr. Snyder. To save time, will members of the panel just raise their right hands if they routinely use retrobulbar anesthesia when using the argon laser. (*None routinely use it.*)

Dr. Zweng. Five percent of the time I need a retrobular to keep the eye steady. (*The panel members agreed.*)

Dr. Okun. We use retrobulbar anesthesia in about 50 percent of the patients on whom we are doing argon laser treatments because a large number of our patients are uniocular (approximately 50 percent) and also because we are frequently coagulating so close to critical structures that the slightest amount of movement of the eye could spell disaster. I have such a movement recorded on our TV camera, with subsequent notching of a major vein. This eye experienced a major vitreous hemorrhage 2 days later. I do not use a retrobulbar in very cooperative patients who can hold their eyes absolutely still.

Dr. Snyder. With certain hand-held fundus contact lenses, can't you control the eye adequately?

Dr. Okun. No, I can't control it adequately. I'm much happier to have the eye absolutely still. From my tone, I think you can tell that I'm not 100 percent happy with argon laser photocoagulation of the disc. The reason for this is that in spite of the most beautiful 24-hour posttreatment pictures that you will ever want to see, 1 to 3 weeks later either these vessels are open once again, or new ones have cropped up. I have patients I have treated nine and ten times, only to have recurrent growth following each attempt. Perhaps 60 to 80 percent of my cases of disc neovascularization are of this type. It is for this reason that I feel that the Zeiss xenon photocoagulator is indispensable in the treatment of all patients who have proliferative diabetic retinopathy, including those with disc neovascularization. Xenon photocoagulation offers the following advantages: (1) all quadrants can be treated at one sitting, (2) most eyes can be treated in spite of early lens changes, and (3) hemorrhages are almost unheard of during treatment.

Only in those patients in whom there is progression of disc neovascularization do I feel it is justified to go ahead with argon laser photocoagulation because, as I stated earlier, the dose which is required to achieve effective permanent occlusion is associated with too high an incidence of serious complications.

Dr. Vaiser. Ed, I would like to know what importance you attribute to fluorescein angiography, mainly in regard to the identification of feeder vessels, and in the treatment of macular edema, and in general its role in photocoagulation of diabetic retinopathy.

Dr. Okun. Let's provoke a little bit of discussion here. I feel that fluorescein is not only not mandatory in all cases but in some instances, the fluorescein injection just prior to treatment may make treatment more difficult because of leakage into the vitreous. In our treatment of macular edema I don't think it makes any difference whatsoever whether or not a previous fluorescein angiogram has been made. If you knock out the things that are red and you stick particularly temporal to the macula, you'll get excellent results.

The only instance where I feel a fluorescein study may be of value is in the treatment of new vessels originating from the disc. In approximately 30 percent of those studied we have been able to identify the feeder vessels; but these cases did not do any better than those in which in which a definite feeder could not be detected. The incidence of recurrence was just as high. However, by avoiding larger collector vessels until later in our treatment session, the incidence of hemorrhage was reduced.

In my experience, identification of feeder vessels is important in helping to avoid hemorrhage, but even when the feeder vessels were closed first, and then the remaining vessels "chopped" up, and repeated hourly, daily, or weekly, this has not affected the recurrence rate. Argon laser treatment is presently resorted to only after definite progression is established following peripapillary and peripheral xenon treatment.

Dr. Snyder. Mort, is it possible that vascular occlusion occurs after 24 hours?

Dr. Goldberg. The sense of the question possibly relates to some of the histologic and electron microscopic material I presented in Chapter 8. Twenty-four hours after argon laser photocoagulation of vessels there was definite necrosis of peri-vascular tissue, but the capillaries and arterioles themselves were remarkably normal. I suppose it is, in fact, possible that long-term observations would show that perivascular inflammation and fibrosis might subsequently squeeze off and obliterate some of the vessels. Apple, Wyhinny, and I have some long-term animal experimentation in progress to settle that point, but we do not have any data available yet. My impression from clinical experience with argon laser photo-coagulation is that if the vessels are not closed at the time of photocoagulation, they are unlikely to close subsequently.

Furthermore, I would agree with Dr. Okun, and would not like him to remain in the minority by himself but would join him in many of his comments, that even if one is able to close neovascular tissue with an argon laser at the time of photo-coagulation, that subsequently the vessels may open up. Thus, one incurs a rather tremendous responsibility for these patients. I, too, have had the unhappy experi-ence of finding myself obligated to re-treat epipapillary neovascular tissue that once was closed and subsequently reopened, as many as nine times; I haven't gone to 10 times yet, but I have had to treat 2 patients nine times. I had been able to close the vessels anteriority to the disc, but when I saw the patients in follow-up, the vessels were open again. Often the vessels increased in size and number, and they often hemorrhaged. I have wished I had never started in these cases, but I have felt obligated to keep on treating them because they appeared to be progressing, perhaps, at least in part, as a result of treatment from photo-coagulation by argon laser.

Dr. Snyder. Is there any work indicating choroidal nonfilling or ischemia of exter-nal retina, such as you have cited in the retinal vasculature?

Dr. Goldberg. There is very little information available. Unfortunately, the indispensable angiographic technique available for the retina, namely fluorescein, is of little value for the choroid unless one is dealing with, let's say, an albino. The few published experiments with choroidal blood flow using fluorescein angiographic techniques were done, in fact, in albinos. Hopefully, with the availability of indocyanine green, so-called cardio-green, and infrared films, it will be possible to visualize the choroidal blood flow by intravenous angiographic techniques. Dr. Patz has had some experience in this area, and perhaps would like to comment on it. I personally have not used this technique as yet.

Dr. Vaiser. Mort, I note that most of your unsuccessful treatments of intraretinal vessels were treated with a 100-μ spot size. Don't you think that a 50-μ spot size might have produced more damage in the vessel and less in the surrounding tissue?

Dr. Goldberg. We have looked at that point fairly carefully in both human and monkey retinas. There is little doubt that the 50-μ spot size, even with wattages as low as 50 and 100 mW for durations of 0.1 and 0.2 seconds, can cause perivascular retinal necrosis and cystoid degeneration without any observable effect on the lumen of the vessel or on the wall of the vessel. I think the spot size, if one compares 50 and 100 μ, is of little significance under these circumstances.

Dr. Vaiser. Hunter, any comments?

Dr. Little. We must have a little rebuttal here after these two previous discussions. First of all I would like to go on record as saying that Dr. Zweng and I own no stock in Coherent Radiation, and we really do not give a damn whether they sell another instrument or not. But I would like to make a few comments relative to the argon. My experience has been that, yes, a large number of these fronds do reopen, and obviously, that is why, as Dr. Okun has said, we have retreated to the ablation because you will knock them out and they'll be beautiful and you'll pat yourself on the back. In some cases I have patted myself on the back so much that I have told the patient I thought we should treat the second eye before she had a hemorrhage. And I have three such patients that actually are now blind. And I think that I had a great deal to do with the progression of their disease course. So I urge you not to treat the second eye, and if you do treat the second eye (I won't say don't do it; I know a great number of people are not doing it—I know Dr. Patz is not doing it) I would wait at least 3 months and preferably 6 months, before treating the second eye, until I can see that first eye has gone through a "quiescent state" without active proliferans. And maybe that's not long enough; but I do know that if you do it sooner than that, you are asking for trouble. I feel very strongly about the importance of fluorescein angiography, if you are going to use argon laser photocoagulation for treating disc vessels. The whole reason to get into this problem of the feeder vessels, etc., was the problem of hemorrhage. We had significant hemorrhages, in the neighborhood of 15 to 20 percent of the cases, and I venture to say that physicians using argon were not getting that much hemorrhage, were really not doing that much to the fronds. But if you go in there and coagulate vessels and obstruct vessels, if you do not do feeder vessel technique, you are going to get hemorrhages in about 15 to 20 percent of your cases. So I think it's mandatory if you are going to take that approach that you get fluorescein pictures. Now, you will not always get the feeder vessel, as I mentioned, but you will find out which vessels not to treat and you will avoid those. Another thing that is extremely important, particularly in treating disc vessels, is that you stay on top of them. You don't just treat them part way and sit tight, you get rid of those vessels; and I agree with Dr. Goldberg that I think if the vessel is not occluded in 24 hours, the chances of it's being occluded in 3 months are about zero. So I think you should stay on top of it and re-treat it until there is nothing there. Once you have accomplished this, I think that, when combined with the ablation, a high percentage of cases, and in my experience thus far 52 percent at 4 to 12 months out, have not had recurrent growth of vessels; whereas, at the end of 4 months, in feeder-frond treatment without 360-degree ablation, over 36 percent had already had recurrent growth of vessels. I'm sure the percentage would be higher if you left them alone and followed them. So if you are going to treat fronds, you have got to eliminate them and I think also if it's an active type frond, you certainly should treat 360 degrees, and that is what I am doing. I find retrobulbar injections not really necessary. I never treat more than 0.1 seconds (50-μ spot 0.1 seconds) and I'll go up from 100 mW at the beginning to 200 to 250 mW; and I caution you, 100 to 150 mW is usually all the power that is necessary if the media are clear. But I think it might be nice to do retrobulbar because you are doing microvascular surgery, you are focusing that 50-μ beam in between vessels and you are nudging in on an area that may be 100 or 200 μ in diameter, and there is a little interplay if you are moving or the patient is moving. But I think you help minimize this by holding the contact lens. A Goldmann lens is one that Dr. Zweng and I prefer rather than the Lo-Vac, where they can move a little bit and you are not holding onto the lens. So, I do not object to the retrobulbar injection, but I just have not found it really necessary in certainly more than 2 to 3 percent of my cases.

Dr. Vaiser. We have been talking until now about the different types of photo-coagulation therapy. I would like to hear Dr. Caird's statistics about patients who have not received any treatment at all, in other words, some comments about the natural history of the disease.

Dr. Caird. An analysis of the data reported at the Airlie House Symposium 4 years ago has been possible.* Each group of lines in Figure 13-1 represents eyes in one retinal category in the O'Hare classification. $N_1F_0H_0$ means that there are less than four areas of new vessels, without fibrous proliferation or preretinal hemorrhage. $N_2F_0H_0$ means four or more, and so on. The eyes are classified by their initial vision as good (G), which means 20/40 or better; impaired (I) means 20/50 to 20/200; and blind (B) means less than 20/200. In the top line are shown eyes in the category $N_1F_1H_0$ with initial good vision; 1 year later only 4 percent are blind. This is very little different from the prognosis for vision in eyes with background retinopathy.† About 14 percent have impaired vision, and the great majority still have good vision 1 year later. This is not too different from some of the results of treatment that we have been told about earlier. With impaired vision, the chance of blindness is higher—20 percent or so in 1 year, but even here there is almost a 20-percent chance of improvement. In category $N_2F_0H_0$ the chance of blindness in 1 year in those with initial good vision is of

* Caird FI, Draper D: Unpublished.

† Caird FI, Garrett CL: Prognosis for vision in diabetic retinopathy. Diabetes 12:389, 1963.

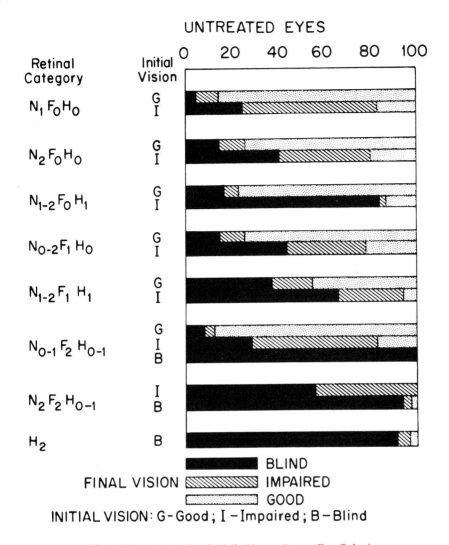

Fig. 13-1.   Analysis of Airlie House Data (Dr. Cairn).

the order of 15 percent, or substantially worse than in category $N_1F_0H_0$; with initial impaired vision it is again substantially worse than the comparable line in the $N_1F_0H_0$ group. Even in the bottom row, (H2) which is preretinal hemorrhage sufficiently severe to prevent classification of the rest of the retina, there is a small but measurable chance of improvement if nothing is done at all. So I think it is important that when thought is being given to consequences of treatment, first, take the initial vision into account and, secondly, remember that even in the worst eyes there is a chance of spontaneous improvement. These, I think are, the two important principles which derive from this. The results in eyes with good vision treated by photocoagulation are identical to those in untreated eyes. This tends, for me at least, to confirm the idea that the stated prognosis for the untreated eyes is correct.

Dr. Vaiser. Ed, any comments?

Dr. Okun. This is a very fine statistical analysis of very poor data. Three months prior to this meeting, participants were told to retrospectively classify their patients. Classification confusion led to the inclusion of background retinopathy with proliferative cases. Second, we are talking about a 1-year follow-up of visual acuity, which depends greatly upon the clarity of the media. That's really very poor in terms of the progression of the retinopathy, because the retinopathy could be going from grade zero to a tremendously involved and advanced stage of retinopathy, as it does, and maintain perfect visual acuity to the last day, when they detach the retina or they get that bad vitreous hemorrhage. So, talking about a 1-year follow-up of patients, and only talking about visual acuity and particularly talking about a group of people who have a retrospective grading of their retinopathy is, I think, a poor way to determine the natural history of the disease process.

Dr. Caird. May I answer the three points? These may be bad data, but at the time they were the only data, and I think this is still the case. Secondly, if the authors who put up the data were muddled, they were all equally muddled, because it is possible to show that the prognosis for vision is the same, if you compare like with like, for at least three groups of investigators contributing enough eyes to make statistical analysis feasible. It seemed that investigators were applying criteria roughly evenly. The same was true for treatment; it didn't seem to matter which ophthalmologist treated you. As far as giving only a 1-year prognosis is concerned, this was all the data would stand. It was necessary to throw out much data where the follow-up was not even 3 months. There was even one set of data, about pituitary ablation, based on the changes in vision that occurred after 10 days; it was said that pituitary ablation was absolutely wonderful.

Dr. Snyder. Any comments, Dr. Kohner?

Dr. Kohner. We do have data on a prospective study which has not yet been fully analyzed. The prospective study was started in 1965 and in this study we took all patients who had mild retinopathy in our diabetic clinic and we followed them by yearly examination, both medically and by retinal photography and visual determination. We found that, of those patients who had no visual symptoms when first seen, 85 percent still had good vision at the end of 5 years. This study was based on approximately 160 eyes and, of these, 85 percent maintained their vision.

Going on to the patients with proliferative retinopathy (and here I must admit that we include intraretinal neovascularization with proliferative retinopathy), provided the patients did not have new vessels on the disc, not more than 1 in 5 patients lost vision, i.e., went from good vision to poor vision, or from good vision to blind in this period of time. I want to emphasize that this is provided they had no vessels on the disc.

Dr. Caird. May I say that the data of Dr. Kohner are very similar to what was published for the first time 10 years ago.* This was based at that time on a 1-year follow-up, but subsequently extended to a 5-year follow-up.†

Dr. Vaiser. Any comments, Dr. Davis?

Dr. Davis. I want to make a comment on the previous discussion between Dr. Okun

---

* Caird FI, Garrett CL: Prognosis for vision in diabetic retinopathy. Diabetes 12:389, 1963.

† Caird FI et al:

and Dr. Little. One factor—and Dr. Zweng and Dr. Little may correct me if they disagree—that perhaps has not been sufficiently emphasized in talking about argon laser photocoagulation is the factor of the rate of blood flow. They mentioned it but I think it bears repeating that the rate of blood flow in the new vessels is very important. As a matter of fact, I have been an advocate of the Lo-Vac flat contact lens for a long time and I didn't really discover until I began using the argon laser photocoagulator that for anything more than a disc diameter half away from the disc, the view one gets with this lens is inferior to that which one gets with the Goldmann no-mirror lens, the reason being that your observation system needs to be almost perpendicular with the front surface of the lens. With the Lo-Vac lens, as you ask the patient to move his eye away from right on the disc or right next to it on the macular side, you begin to get distortion because your view is no longer perpendicular to the front surface of the lens. With the Goldmann lens, the eye turns behind the lens and you can stay perpendicular.

I should have figured that out 15 years ago, but I didn't figure it out until, looking through the argon laser slit-lamp photocoagulator delivery system, it became clear to me that it was so critical to know whether you are treating on the arteriole side or the venous side. If you are treating new vessels directly, all of a sudden it came like a bolt from the blue that I had to have better visualization. And I think that is largely what Dr. Little is saying when he emphasizes fluorescein. I think that is part of this disagreement about retrobulbar or no.

Now, again, I hope someone will raise his hand and correct me if he thinks that I am too complacent about treating over the disc and over large vessels. But in my experience the very rapid flow of the normal retinal vessels over the disc is such that it is very hard to make one of those big vessels bleed, unless your power is very excessive. And I think it is possible, if you treat arterial feeders first and slow the flow down, that you can then treat with a good deal of safety even though there is a little motion. You can treat the new vessels because the power level at which you are treating is such that you will not do much to the large vessels because in them the blood flow is still so rapid that you have the radiator cooling effect. I did not want to let this discussion go by without emphasizing that, in my opinion, you must see fairly well to treat focally with argon, and I use this example of the contact lens because, as I say, I had been using the flat contact lens for 10 years, thinking it was great, but I was not using argon laser to treat new vessels focally during that time. I think it's very important for any of you who may have just started using an argon to realize that you really need to see what you are doing. As I believe Dr. L'Esperance said, the xenon arc machine is very forgiving of the operator's lack of precision.

Dr. Vaiser. What type of contact lens are you using in conjunction with the argon laser? Also, I would like you to comment on the importance of fluorescein angiography in the treatment of macular edema.

Dr. Zweng. I couldn't agree more that the beam must be focused carefully and that the Goldmann macular contact lens is the lens of choice in the posterior pole; and it is the one that we use all of the time for treating the posterior pole. I too have been recently reintroduced to the concept of peripheral astigmatism in getting some material out of Rhesus monkeys to show the different spot sizes, from 50 μ up to 1000 μ. I got just a little off axis with the 500-μ spot-size lesion and, of course, it was a slight elipse—it was not perfectly round. And also the focusing front and back has to be done very carefully and very precisely. But if one does that, of course he is rewarded by higher yield of closures that last longer than a couple of hours. I do wish to make a couple of other comments about things that have come up in the meantime. For a little over 6 months I have been using just the peripheral ablative technique; it is quite widespread and quite complete. I have yet to have my first instance of bleeding of the nerve head in the immediate postoperative period. Dr. Little had 1 case; I wonder if it was not a case of post hoc ergo propter hoc, that is, a coincidence; because as I say, I do not know exactly how many I have treated, but it must be somewhere from 60 to 75, and not one has bled from those new blood vessels off the nerve head. Of course, we carefully caution the patients to be gentle with themselves.

Finally, I would like to talk about fluorescein angiography and macular edema. I cannot agree with Dr. Okun that fluorescein angiography is not necessary in treating macular edema, and that if you treat everything that is red, you get it all.

Recently, in perhaps the last 2 months, when I was in doubt about the angiogram, I stained carefully and, looking at the macula with the contact lens and all under the slit lamp, I gave the patient an injection of fluorescein (we have a modification on our slit lamp which lets us insert a cobalt blue filter and also we have a 50-W bulb which, again, Coherent Radiation should retrofit every unit with). Then, watching the dye go through and then going back and forth between the cobalt blue filter and the white light, the leaking point, as demonstrated by fluorescein angioscopy, often is not associated with a red spot. There is some intraretinal leakage area that needs to be photocoagulated that I would have missed had I just used red as the basis for treatment.

Dr. Goldberg. I'd like to ask you why you stopped treating the disc itself and why are you limiting yourself to peripheral argon treatment rather than this combined assault on the disc. Were there complications of argon laser photocoagulation on the disc itself?

Dr. Zweng. Sure, we had complications, as Dr. Little said, about a 15 percent hemorrhage rate. I think originally we were quite bemused by our seeming ability to stop or interrupt blood flow, and you can certainly interrupt blood flow without too much trouble in the collector vessels. They are larger, the flow is slower. If you want to look very good in front of someone who is watching you through the stovepipe, you can just go over a collecting vessel and that will usually obliterate very promptly. It's those feeder vessels that are narrow and their flow therefore faster that are the challenge. We did have too high a hemorrhage rate because we were treating those collecting vessels; meanwhile blood was still going into the frond, and finally there was so much that there would be a hemorrhage, either as we watched, or the next day. So, what to do? Dr. Little and Dr. Patz conceived the idea of the feeder vessel treatment. But it also seemed that when we treated some patients with xenon arc with widespread retinal disease who also had nerve head neovascularization, there was a quite striking reduction in neovascularization. So I think that possibly the failures that have been encountered with xenon arc photocoagulation using the peripheral ablative technique involve still having neovascularization on the nerve head—in fact, progressing; I think possibly—this is an hypothesis—it was not done adequately, or fully enough. As I said before, there must be atrophy of the nerve head, and one of the reasons is not only the periphery but also the pathology in the macula needs to be treated, and also in the macular papillary bundle which you said we can do with an argon photocoagulation. But I went to this because I want to see if this technique done in this way will not give the result we want, not only just for now, but also to protect the patient against the future retinopathy.

Dr. Goldberg. Even with feeder vessel technique we have unfortunately experienced a rather high complication rate by treating immediately on the disc, that is, treating epipapillary neovascular tissue. Not only have those complications included hemorrhage, but also central scotomas, permanent central scotomas in 2 cases, unfortunately, and occlusion of a peripapillary arteriole with a permanent absolute sector defect.

Dr. Snyder. I have a question for Dr. Siperstein. If diabetes mellitus is inherited as recessive, why do you expect only 75 percent of the offsprings to be diabetic, that is, if both parents have the disease? I calculate 100-percent incidence in this circumstance.

Dr. Siperstein. You are absolutely correct. The calculated incidence should be 100 percent if the individuals one is following live long enough. The problem in documenting 100-percent penetrance of any genes involves extrapolations to ages 70 and 80 and, of course, not everyone being followed lives so long. But theoretically, if one has complete penetrance of the recessive gene, 100 percent of the offspring of two diabetic parents should develop the lesion. With the electron microscopic detection of capillary basement membrane thickening, we think we will approach that figure long before age 60 to 70 because hyperglycemia, as I implied, seems to be a late complication of diabetes mellitus.

Dr. Goldberg. In Figure 13-2 a red-free view of the disc is seen prior to argon

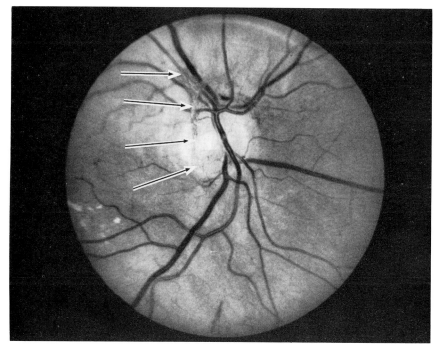

Fig. 13-2. Red-free view of disc showing fine neovascular tissue (arrows) (cf. Figs. 13-3, 13-4, 13-5 and 13-6).

laser photocoagulation, and some fine neovascular tissue can be seen (arrows). Several weeks after argon laser photocoagulation, Figure 13-3 shows not only an increase in the number of new blood vessels on the disc but a spontaneous linear hemorrhage (arrow). At this point we felt obliged to re-treat again. Now, treating only with intensity sufficient to just induce spasm of the neovascular tissue and using a feeder vessel technique, marked swelling of the disc can be seen 12 hours after photocoagulation (Fig. 13-4). Figure 13-5 indicates that there is no major macular vessel occlusion to account for what is seen in Figure 13-6, namely, a dense central scotoma which has persisted for 10 months, dropping visual acuity from 20/20 to 20/400. I think it is important to stress this type of complication, even though it is uncommon, because it is held in the literature and numerous places that the safest place to use an argon laser is immediately on the disc. I would hope you would conclude from this uncommon complication, as well as from the histologic material and electron microscopic material (Chapter 8), that the disc parenchyma and the nerve fiber layer of the retina are not immune to therapeutic levels of argon laser photocoagulation.

Dr. Vaiser. Hunter, could we hear from you regarding complications encountered with the use of the argon laser?

Dr. Little. We have had several nerve fiber field defects. Dr. Goldberg, it looked like you were treating a previously treated area. Figure 13-7 is a little diagram showing complications of argon laser photocoagulation which, incidentally, we could not get on the Academy program because there was not sufficient interest in the subject, according to the reviewer. Nevertheless, on your left, before photocoagulation the retina is about 1 mm thick whereas on the right, after photocoagulation, you will note that the retina is markedly thin, the nerve fiber layer is much closer to the pigment epithelial layer, and there has been hyperplasia of the retinal pigment epithelial layer. So we will get greater absorption of the light by the increased pigment epithelium; and since the nerve fiber layer is closer to this pigment, you are going to get more heat. So, the problem is in repeated coagulation in the peripapillary area, where one is in danger of severe trouble in producing a nerve fiber field defect. And if the patient is, say, myopic or has some other reason to have atrophy in the peripapillary area, I think he too might be more susceptible to this problem. Another case illustrates a complication from very heavy photocoagulation over the disc. In a young diabetic with proliferans off the disc this complication occurred after we got the commercially available laser where we had much greater power than we had previously with the N.I.H. photo type model. For the first time we could identify knocking out all kinds of vessels, but to do this I used a large spot size and just sort of indiscriminately treated the whole frond. The patient returned the day after treatment and couldn't see my hand. He had ischemic papillitis or thermal papillitis from heavy coagulation. And the point is, if you are going to treat such cases with disc vessels, use a small spot size, 50 μ or 100 μ, but never go up to 500 μ with high powers or you will destroy too much nerve tissue. The peripapillary area is most dangerous, particularly in re-treatment. For treating the disc, treat the vessel, not the disc.

One other complication that should be mentioned is corneal burns. You can get corneal burns with the argon laser if you use a 100-μ spot size with powers over, say, 300 or 400 mW. The reason is that, with the 100-μ spot setting, the beam is small at the level of the cornea.

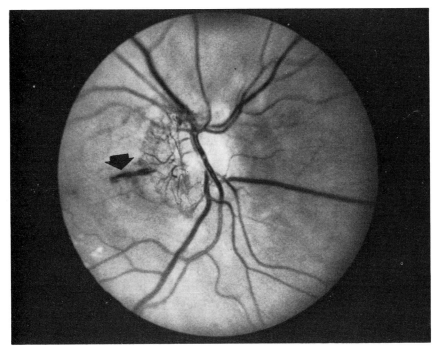

Fig. 13-3. Several weeks after argon laser treatment there are an increased number of new blood vessels on the disc and a spontaneous hemorrhage (arrow) (cf. Figs. 13-2, 13-4, 13-5 and 13-6).

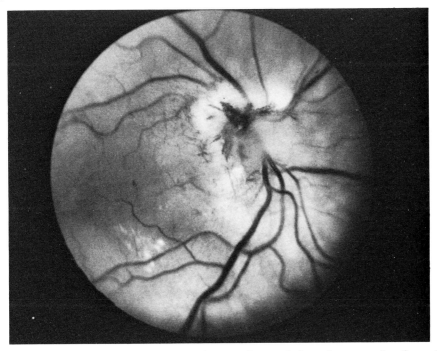

Fig. 13-4. Twelve hours after feeder vessel coagulation of neovascular tissue (cf. Figs. 13-2, 13-3, 13-5 and 13-6).

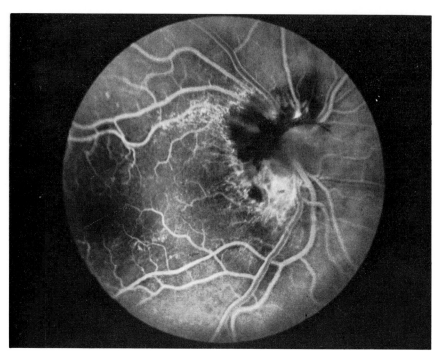

Fig. 13-5. Fluorescein angiogram indicating no major macular vessel occlusion to account for dense central scotoma seen in Fig. 13-6 (cf. Fig. 13-2, 13-3 and 13-4).

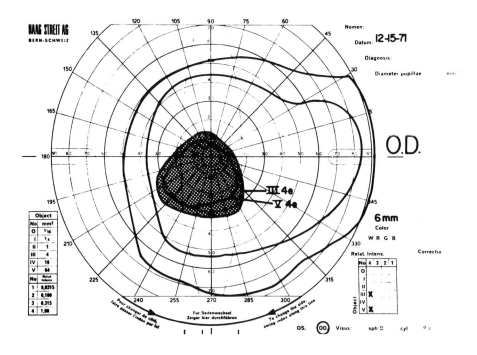

Fig. 13-6. Central scotoma after disc coagulation with argon laser. Visual acuity has dropped from 20/20 to 20/400 (cf. Figs. 13-2, 13-3, 13-4 and 13-5).

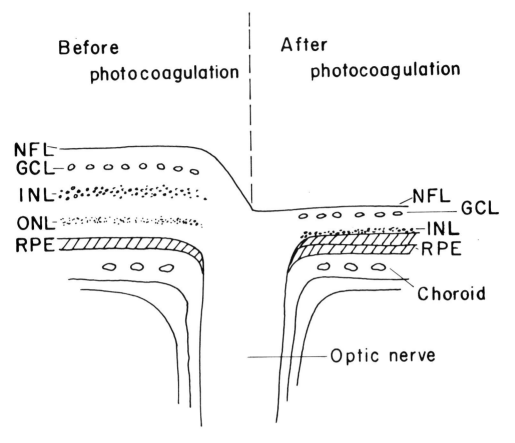

Fig. 13-7. Diagram illustrates close proximity of nerve fiber layer to hyperplastic retinal epithelium in scarred retina repeat photocoagulation about the optic disc. (Reprinted with permission from Little HL, Zweng HC: Complications of argon laser retinal photocoagulation. 1971 Transactions of the Pacific Coast Oto-Ophthalmological Society.)

Dr. Goldberg. I suspect strongly that what Dr. Little said is absolutely correct and that his advice is well taken. When one re-treats over a previously treated area, the heat producing pigment epithelium is certainly closer to the nerve fiber layer. One might, in these circumstances, induce central or other field defects. The same is true of a previously *untreated* area, as we have shown. Even if one treats around the disc and around the macula, where the nerve fiber layer is extremely thick, with burns of clinical intensity, it is still possible to cause necrosis of the nerve fiber layer, even if there has not been previous treatment. The particular case I illustrated never did have peripapillary treatment; it was all done immediately on the disc itself.

Gholam A. Peyman
Morton F. Goldberg

Chapter 14
Surgical Treatment of Vitreous Hemorrhage

Vitreous hemorrhage in the course of diabetic retinopathy often is the final step toward blindness. This catastrophic episode brings with it psychological, economic, and social consequences for the patient and his family. The uncertainty about reabsorption and treatment of vitreous hemorrhage is well known to all ophthalmologists. The serious prognosis for visual function in diabetic retinopathy was evaluated by Caird and Garret in 1963.[1] In fact, one-third of their patients suffering from vitreous hemorrhage became blind only 1 year after the initial hemorrhagic episode. Blindness is caused mainly by the opacities which form in the vitreous if the blood does not reabsorb. Band and membrane formation also may complicate this condition, leading to tractional detachment of the retina. In addition, the large amount of iron discharged from hemoglobin can cause degeneration of the retina.

Although surgical treatment of vitreous hemorrhage does not attack the basic cause of the disease, it can nevertheless be very rewarding in terms of the immediate visual function of the patient. Removal of vitreous opacities after vitreous hemorrhage has been advocated for about a century.[2, 3] However, lack of proper instrumentation has prevented the procedure from becoming a clinical reality.

INSTRUMENTATION

During the past year we have developed the necessary instrumentation for vitrectomy, including (1) an instrument for cutting, removing and replacing vitreous (vitrophage),[4, 5] (2) a slit illuminator for use with the operating microscope for intravitreal surgery,[6] and (3) a micromanipulator arc system for accurate manipulation inside the eye.[7] Other centers have developed similar instrumentation.[8, 9, 10]

Vitrophage

The cutting apparatus of this instrument consists of two concentric tubes. The outer tube has two openings at the distal end. The one closer to the tip is used for suction; the second opening, 180 degrees opposite the first and further

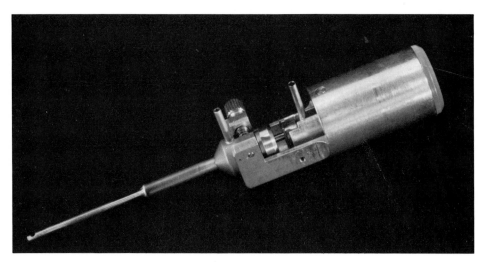

Fig. 14-1. Vitrophage.

from the tip, is used as an infusion port (Figs. 14-1 and 14-2). Cutting is performed by the spring-loaded sharp end of the inner tube oscillating against the distal opening of the outer tube. Opaque vitreous cut by the blade is removed through the inner tube by suction. The infusion and suction is regulated by a system of push-and-pull syringes,[1] thus achieving an equal amount of infusion and suction. The linear oscillation of the inner tube is performed by an air-pressure-driven system located at the proximal end of the instrument. This system in turn is connected to a pulse generator which regulates pulsation frequency (Fig. 14-3). The latter can be regulated from one time per 10 seconds to five times per second.

(A movie was shown to demonstrate the cutting action of the vitrophage in experimentally induced vitreous opacities in a sheep's eye.)

Visualization

Currently available operating microscopes do not provide a light source capable of illumination at the variety of depths and angles necessary for precise instrumentation during intraocular procedures. While the conventional slit lamp

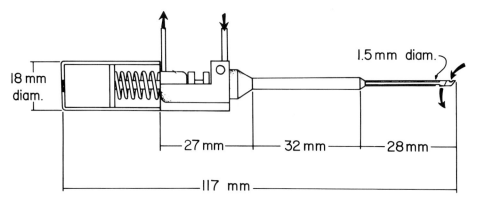

Fig. 14-2. Schematic diagram of vitrophage and its dimensions.

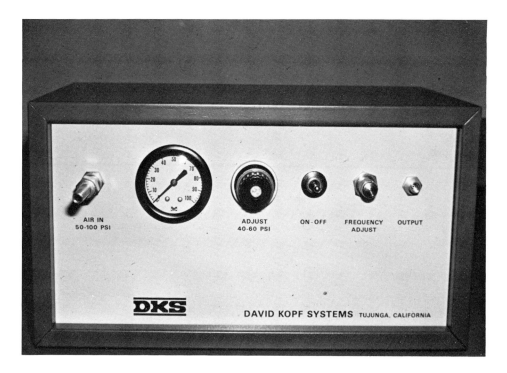

Fig. 14-3.   Control system for air pressure pulsation.

provides proper visualization of the vitreous body and fundus when the patient is sitting, this type of illumination has not been used with the patient in the supine position.

The illumination system which we have developed [6] employs a conventional slit source of illumination from a slit-lamp microscope mounted on a Zeiss operating microscope via an arc-shaped track (Fig. 14-4). The track provides movement of the illuminator from 30 degrees right azimuth through the coaxial position to 30 degrees left azimuth (Fig. 14-5). We have chosen 200 mm as a convenient operating distance. The track has been designed so that the slit illuminator revolves at the focal point of the objective lens of the operating microscope. Our system renders all the quality of the conventional slit lamp but can be used with the patient in a horizontal position.

Micromanipulator Arc System

Intravitreal surgery is a particularly difficult ophthalmologic procedure because of the small space available within the eye for manipulation of the instruments. Even a slight miscalculation or unsteady motion could injure the delicate surrounding structures, i.e., the lens and retina. To provide control and add a "second pair of hands," we have developed the micromanipulator arc system.[7] This system consists of a support platform and head rest, vertical and horizontal gross adjustment controls, and the instrument holder. The instrument to be used in the intraocular procedure (e.g., the vitrophage) is inserted into the instrument holder on the arc (Fig. 14-6). The in-and-out movement into the vitreous cavity is

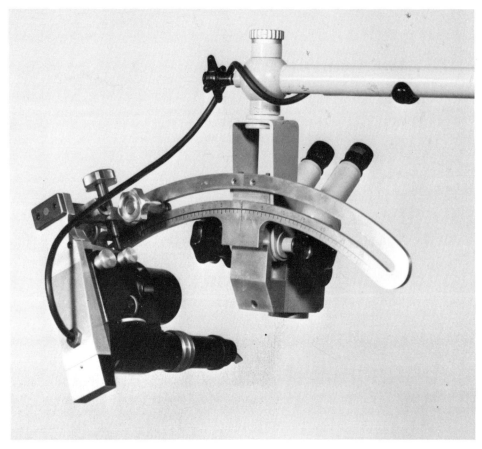

Fig. 14-4. Slit illuminator mounted on a narc track behind the Zeiss operating microscope.

achieved by means of a variable angle adjustable rod; turning a hand-nut inserts or retracts the instrument. The angle of insertion is varied by a rack-and-pinion mechanism which moves the instrument along the arc-shaped track (Fig. 14-7). The track is mounted to the rest of the system by means of a pivot-joint which permits 360-degree rotation of the arc about the horizontal radius (Fig. 14-8). The combination of movements permits the tip of the instrument to reach a cone-shaped area inside the eye, while the position of the instrument at the sclerotomy site (center of the arc) remains stable. This system permits controlled movements of an instrument inside the vitreous body.

INDICATIONS FOR VITRECTOMY

Many diseases of the retinal circulatory system can lead to vitreous hemorrhage, such as diabetic retinopathy, Eales' disease, sickle cell disease, and venous occlusion. Proliferative diabetic retinopathy is the most frequently encountered cause. The degree of cloudiness of the vitreous in vitreous hemorrhage depends first on the amount of bleeding and second on the prehemorrhagic condition of the vitreous. Whereas a small amount of bleeding often remains localized in a

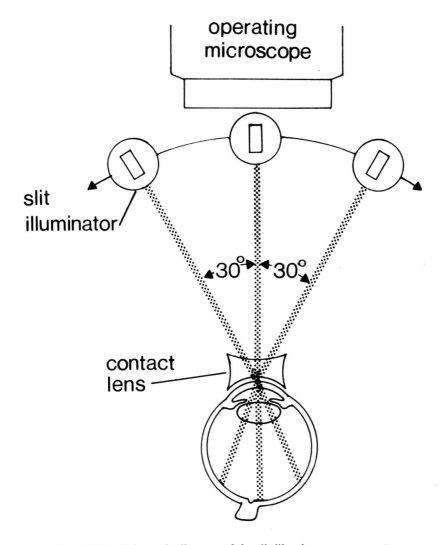

Fig. 14-5.   Schematic diagram of the slit illuminator movements.

healthy vitreous, it can cause moderate cloudiness in a liquified or posteriorly
detached vitreous. Minute to moderate amounts of bleeding can often become
reabsorbed. However, a repeated or massive vitreous hemorrhage is less likely
to clear completely.

Our indications for vitrectomy have thus far been limited to severe vitreous
hemorrhage with at least 6 months' duration and reduced visual acuity to less
than 20/200. These criteria are not yet standardized, and each case should be
evaluated separately.

Prior to vitrectomy, electroretinogram (ERG) and ultrasound examinations
are performed in addition to the routine ophthalmologic examination. An eye with
a completely extinguished ERG has minimal likelihood of an improvement in
visual acuity even after successful vitrectomy. The ultrasound recording must
also be evaluated carefully, as a membrane formation in the vitreous can simulate

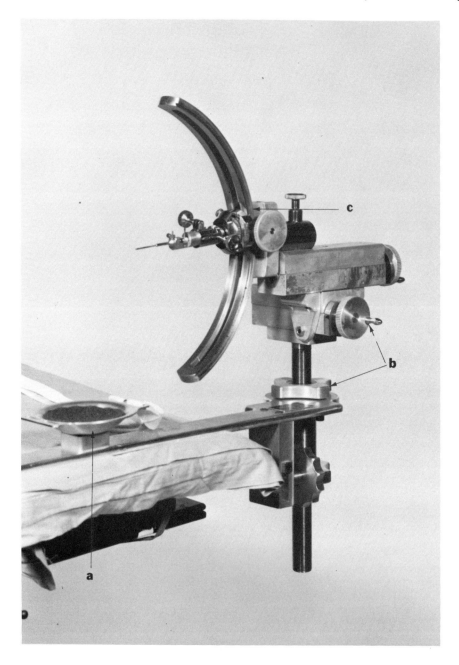

Fig. 14-6. Micromanipulator arc system: (a) head holder; (b) horizontal and vertical gross adjustment controls and (c) arc and instrument holder.

retinal detachment. Nonetheless, if ultrasound reveals a significant retinal detachment posterior to the vitreous hemorrhage, vitrectomy is generally not done. Vitrectomy may, however, be useful in some cases of retinal detachment caused by dense, strong vitreous bands and membranes.

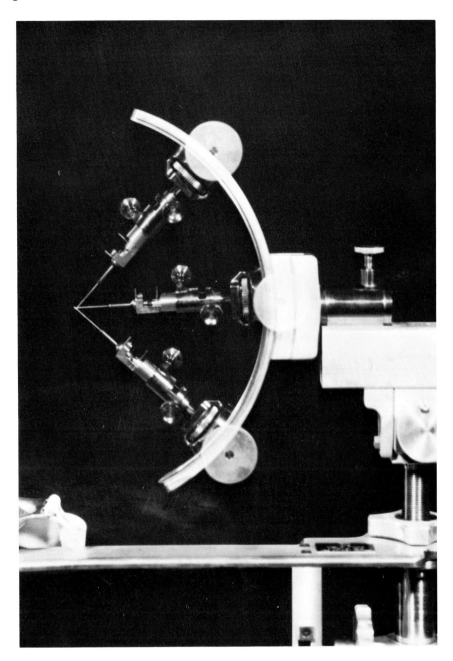

Fig. 14-7. Micromanipulator system showing rack-and-pinion motion. Note that the insertion point at the sclerotomy site remains stationary during rack-and-pinion motion. (Multiple film exposure to demonstrate motion.)

OPERATIVE TECHNIQUE

In the patients operated thus far, we have utilized both the "open sky" and pars plana techniques. The degree of lens opacity has led us to choose one or the other method.

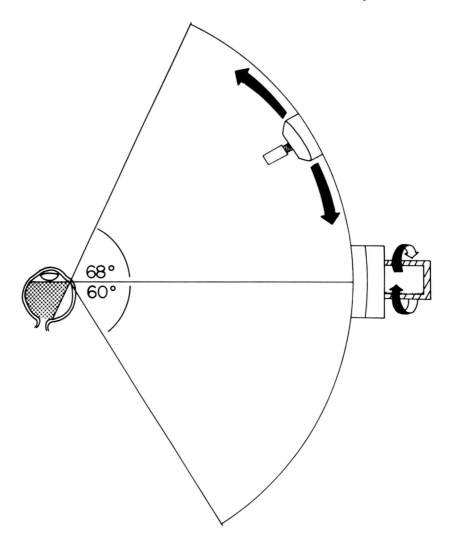

Fig. 14-8. Schematic diagram of micromanipulator system showing the rotational motions of the arc.

Open Sky Method

This technique is performed on patients with significant vitreous hemorrhage and moderate lens opacities requiring cataract extraction. Our technique of corneal incision and cataract extraction is basically similar to Kasner's technique,[11] but with some modifications. We perform a large canthotomy and apply tractional sutures to the lids. After a complete separation of the conjunctiva, a Flieringa ring is sutured to the sclera by a continuous interlocking 6.0 silk suture. Then, two tractional sutures are run beneath the superior and inferior recti and locked with the Flieringa ring and retracted to the forehead and cheek (Fig. 14-9). This maneuver relieves the pressure points beneath the muscles and brings the eye into a slightly exophthalmic position. Then, a 200-degree corneal incision is made at the limbus using a Bard-Parker knife and a corneal scissors. The incision is

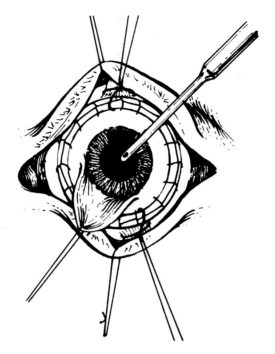

Fig. 14-9. Schematic diagram of the eye. Note fixation ring and sutures in open sky surgery with vitrophage.

made in such a fashion that the attached portion of the cornea lies in the inferonasal quadrant (Fig. 14-9). The corneal flap is then retracted by a 6.0 silk suture. The cataract extraction and a large sector iridectomy at the 12 o'clock position are performed routinely. Our technique differs from Kasner's method in that we do not use the "Weck" sponge and scissors for vitrectomy. With the vitrophage, vitrectomy can be performed with an operating microscope through the dilated pupil. The central portion of deformed vitreous is removed and replaced continuously with normal saline, thus creating a clear tunnel in the visual axis running from the central portion of the fundus to the pupil. After the vitrectomy is performed, the corneal wound is resutured with 9-0 nylon sutures. During the procedure the cornea is protected from drying by a gelatin cup and intermittent irrigation with normal saline.

Pars Plana Technique

This route is chosen in aphakic patients or those with clear lenses. The fixation of the eye is similar to the open sky technique except that we use a special contact lens holder (Figs. 14-10 and 14-11) instead of a Flieringa ring. The contact lens can be inserted into the contact lens holder, thus eliminating the need for holding the lens during the procedure. The operation is performed under direct observation of the fundus with an operating microscope, using the described slit illumination system and a low-vacuum contact lens. A 3-mm meridional sclerotomy is performed at the pars plana on the temporal side of the eye. Two 5-0 nylon sutures are placed over the sclerotomy, which is then surrounded by diathermy applications. The vitrophage mounted on the micro-

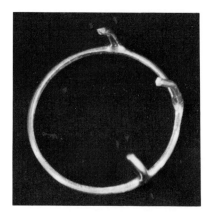

Fig. 14-10.   Contact lens support ring.

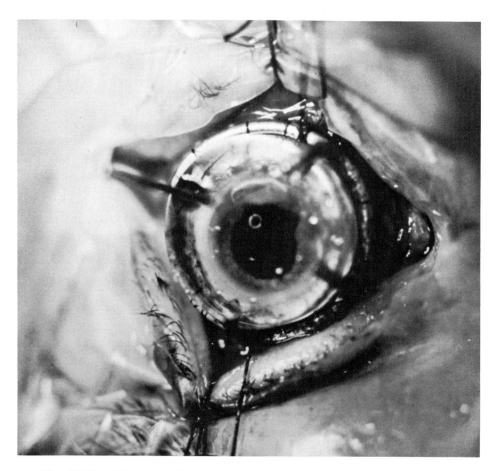

Fig. 14-11.   Photograph showing the technique of eye fixation for the pars plana approach. Note that the eye is fixed in position by two tractional sutures attached to the contact lens holder and superior and inferior recti.

manipulator arc system is then adjusted for the insertion. Prior to the insertion, the eyewall at the site of the sclerotomy is perforated with a sharp knife. The vitrophage is immediately inserted into the eye, and one of the sutures are pulled tightly around the vitrophage tip and tied. The operation is done under observation through the microscope at 25 magnifications. In this procedure, as in the open sky technique, only the central portion of the diseased vitreous is removed and replaced with saline (Figs. 14-12 and 14-13 in the color section), thereby creating a clear tunnel in the visual axis. Figure 14-13 shows an aphakic eye after pars plana vitrectomy.

COMPLICATIONS

In our limited experience with humans we have not encountered any complications during the procedure. This does not mean that they may not occur in subsequent cases. Pulling and tearing the retina is possible if too strong suction is applied to the vitreous. However, the actual cutting of the vitreous bands and opacities with the vitrophage does not cause shearing of the vitreous fibers because the motion of the oscillatory system stops 0.5 mm below the distal opening. This oscillatory principle eliminates the danger of wrapping the vitreous fibers around the inner tube as might occur with a rotary system. Direct injury of the lens and retina by the instrument can also occur. However, the potential for this complication has been reduced to a minimum by proper visualization of the fundus with the slit illuminator. After open sky surgery some post operative corneal edema and opacities have been observed. This complication can be attributed to mechanical injury or drying of the corneal endothelium during the procedure. To prevent corneal opacification in open sky surgery, at the present time we utilize a corneal protector. The corneal flap is kept in the patient's serum during the surgery and is resutured with a continuous 9-0 nylon.[12]

ACKNOWLEDGMENTS

We thank David Kopf Company for assistance in designing and construction of vitrophage, George Merz and Alfred Nelken in construction of slit illumination system and micromanipulator, and Helen Silver for photographic assistance.

REFERENCES

1. Caird FI, Garret CL: Prognosis for vision in diabetic retinopathy. Diabetes 12:389, 1963
2. Ford V: Proposed surgical treatment of opaque vitreous. Lancet 1:462, 1890
3. Peyman GA, May DR, Ericson ES: Techniques of vitreous removal. Survey Ophthalmol 17:29, 1972
4. Peyman GA, Dodich NA: Experimental vitrectomy; instrumentation and surgical technique. Arch Ophthalmol 86:548, 1971
5. Peyman GA, Daily MJ, Ericson ES: Experimental vitrectomy, new technical aspects. Am J Ophthalmol 75:774, 1973
6. Peyman GA, Ericson ES, May DR: Slit illumination system and contact lens support ring for use with operating microscope. Ophthal Surg. 3:29, 1972
7. Peyman GA, Ericson ES, May DR: Micromanopulator arc system for intravitreal surgery. Am J Ophthalmol 75:706, 1973
8. Machemer R, Buettner H, Norton EWD, Parel JM: Vitrectomy: A pars plana approach. Trans Am Acad Ophthalmol Otolaryngol 75:813, 1971
9. Freeman HM: Vitreous surgery. X. Current status of vitreous surgery in cases of rhegmatogenous retinal detachment. Trans Am Acad Ophthalmol Otolaryngol 77:OP-202, 1973

10. Straatsma BR, Griffin JR, Kreiger AE: Stereotaxic intraocular surgery; use in vitreous and posterior segment surgery. Arch Opthalmol 88:325, 1972

11. Kasner D: Personal interview: Vitrectomy: A new approach to the management of vitreous. Highlights Ophthalmol 11:304, 1969

12. Peyman GA, Crouch EJ: Prevention of Corneal opacification in open sky vitrectomy. Ann Ophthamol (in press)

Eva M. Kohner

Chapter 15
A Controlled Trial of Pituitary Ablation

Marked improvement in some features of diabetic retinopathy occurs on occasions following pituitary ablation (Figs. 15-1 and 15-2). If all the results were as striking as the one illustrated, the operation would be justified without further

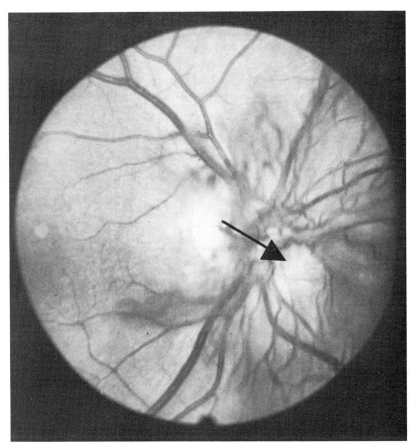

Fig. 15-1. Right disc of patient with many new vessels. *Arrow* points at small area of retinitis proliferans (cf. Fig. 15-2).

This work was supported by the Wellcome Trust and the Scientific Section of The British Diabetic Association.

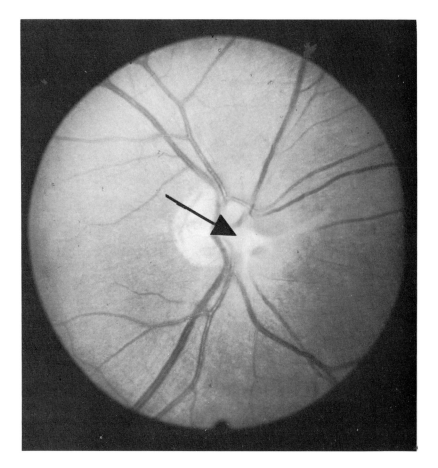

Fig. 15-2. Same patient as Figure 15-1 but 2 years after complete ablation of the pituitary gland. New vessels have regressed and only a small area of retinitis proliferans remains (*arrow*). Note also reduction in diameter of main vessels.

argument. Since, however, some workers find that pituitary ablation does not influence diabetic retinopathy,[1] it is important to have strictly controlled clinical trials to define the place of pituitary ablation in the management of diabetic retinopathy.

This paper reports on such a randomized study, which was carried out in the Hammersmith Hospital, London, between January 1, 1965 and December 31, 1969.

It is important to emphasize these dates since clearly the criteria for inclusion into the study and details of the protocol were laid down in 1964, i.e., at a time when our knowledge about diabetic retinopathy was considerably less than it is today.

PATIENTS AND METHODS

Patients with diabetic retinopathy referred for pituitary ablation entered the trial if they fulfilled the following criteria:

1. They had visual sypmtoms related to the retinopathy and were anxious to have treatment for it.
2. They had at least one eye which had lesions considered to be treatable or reversible by pituitary ablation. Such an eye had to have a visual actuity of 20/80 or better. It was essential that the macula of this eye should not be threatened by fibrous retinitis proliferans and/or retinal detachment.
3. The severity of the retinopathy had to be between certain lower and upper limits.

The lower limits for new vessels were defined as at least grade 2 of the Hammersmith grading system in at least two photographic fields (Fig. 15-3), and for microaneurysms and hemorrhages, at least two photographic fields had to have lesions as severe as those illustrated in Figure 15-4.

It is important to emphasize that the presence of new vessels was not absolutely essential for inclusion into the trial because in 1964 we did not realize that in the absence of proliferative lesions, microaneurysms and hemorrhages had a good prognosis.

The upper limit of new vessels is shown in Figure 15-5. Any patient who had new vessels in excess of these and whose eye was still treatable was

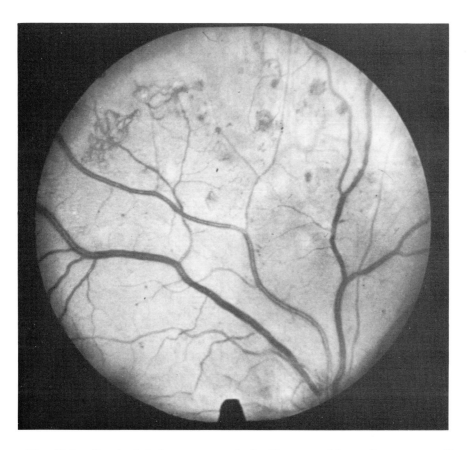

Fig. 15-3. Standard 2 for new vessels in Hammersmith grading system (Reprinted with permission from Oakley et al: Diabetologia 3:402, 1962).

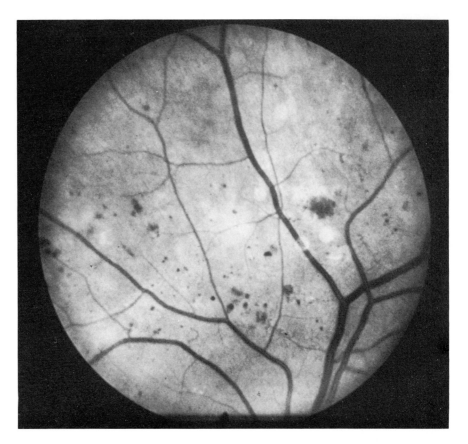

Fig. 15-4. Standard 3 for hemorrhages and microaneurysms in Hammersmith grading system (Reprinted with permission from Oakley et al: Diabetologia 4:202, 1967).

    offered pituitary ablation without randomization since it was known that untreated the prognosis for these eyes was poor and they were the ones most likely to respond to complete pituitary ablation.

4. The general health of the patient had to be adequate. In particular, patients with blood urea over 75 mg/100 ml were excluded, as were patients with angina, past history of myocardial infarction, and symptoms of cerebral and peripheral vascular disease.

5. The referring physician had to be agreeable to the randomization.

    Patients who fulfilled these criteria were allocated into treatment or control groups by a random procedure. Pituitary ablation was performed through trans-sphenoidal yttrium-90 implantation aiming at 150,000 rads to the gland periphery. Both groups were seen at regular intervals, approximately three-monthly in the first year and six-monthly thereafter. The follow-up included at least yearly medical examination, retinal photographs, and visual acuity determination.

    The retinopathy features were analyzed, component by component, using standard photographs for comparison. This gave a numerical grading for each retinopathy feature which allowed for statistical analysis. The method was de-

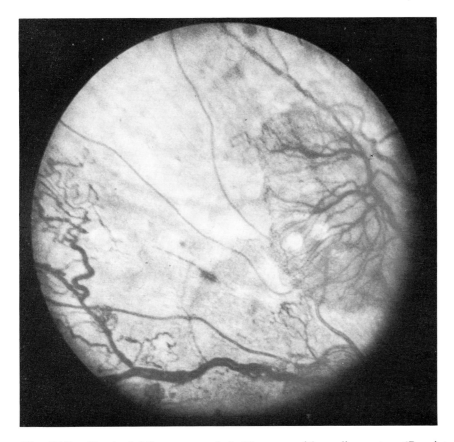

Fig. 15-5. Standard 3 for new vessels in Hammersmith grading system (Reprinted with permission from Oakley et al: Diabetologia 3:402, 1967).

scribed by Oakley et al.[2] Since some patients had two treatable eyes and some only one, and it was the patient who was randomized, in those patients with two treatable eyes the mean figure for the two eyes was taken for each retinopathy feature.

RESULTS

The results will be discussed under four headings: (1) initial assessment; (2) mortality; (3) response of retinopathy features; and (4) response of visual acuity.

Initial Assessment

There were 26 patients with 37 treatable eyes in the pituitary-ablated group and 26 patients with 39 treatable eyes in the control group.

The medical characteristics of the two groups were similar (Table 15-1). They were comparable concerning age, duration of diabetes, and number requiring insulin. The blood pressure and blood urea levels too were similar.

The mean grading for the individual retinopathy features was similar in all respects (Table 15-2) except for the new vessels. In this, the most important

Table 15-1
Randomly Selected Pituitary Implant and Control Patients

	Mean ± S.E.	
	Implant	*Control*
No. of patients	26	26
Age (years)	41.0 ± 2	42.9 ± 2.2
Duration of diabetes (years)	17.2 ± 2	17.8 ± 9.2
No. requiring insulin	19	19
Initial blood urea (mg/100 ml)	38.2 ± 2.2	38.7 ± 4.7
Initial systolic B.P.	143.8 ± 3.7	144.6 ± 4.7
Initial diastolic B.P.	85.7 ± 1.9	86.0 ± 2.8

parameter, the pituitary-ablated group had significantly worse grading, thus indicating poorer prognosis.

Further analysis of the new vessels showed that 10 eyes of the control patients and 5 of the treated patients were free of new vessels. Furthermore, 25 eyes of pituitary ablated patients and 20 eyes of the controls had new vessels on the disc, emphasizing further the poorer prognosis for vision in the pituitary-ablated group.

Mortality

Table 15-3 shows the mortality in the two groups. There were 6 patients who died in the pituitary-ablated group, and 2 in the control series. Of the 6 pituitary-ablated patients, the death of 2 was directly related to the operation. One had CSF rhinorrhea and became unconscious following severe headache at home. His death may have been due to steroid deficiency. The second patient developed meningitis 6 weeks postoperatively. He inhaled vomit while recovering, and died shortly thereafter. The other 4 patients died in the fourth postoperative year, so their deaths cannot be attributed to the operation. Nevertheless, the number of patients who died after the operation is significantly higher than in the control group. This may indicate that the hypopituitary state makes patients less resistant to the vascular disease from which diabetics suffer. It must be emphasized that this death rate is no higher than that reported by Deckert and his

Table 15-2
Initial Eye Assessment of Randomly Selected Pituitary-Implant and Control Patients.

	Mean ± S.E.		
	Implant	*P*	*Control*
Visual Acuity	2.11 ± 0.25 (2 = 6/)	N.S.	1.81 ± 0.24 (1 = 6/)
Microaneurysms and Hemorrhages	2.06 ± 0.21	N.S.	1.93 ± 0.10
New Vessels	1.77 ± 0.15	< 0.01	1.10 ± 0.14
Retinitis Proliferans	0.94 ± 0.21	N.S.	1.16 ± 0.23
Hard Exudates	0.91 ± 0.23	N.S.	1.07 ± 0.15

Table 15-3
Randomly Selected Implant and Control Patients

		Implant	Control
No. died		6	2
No. died due to implant		2	—
Initial blood urea in those who died:	50.8 mg/100 ml		
		p < 0.01	
Initial blood urea in those alive:	36.9 mg/100 ml		

co-workers [3] in untreated young diabetics with proliferative retinopathy.

Comparing the initial blood urea in those patients who died and those who stayed alive, it is seen to be significantly higher in the former. Higher blood urea is thus associated with increased mortality. Largely as a result of these findings, we now only offer pituitary ablation to those whose blood urea is under 50 mg/100 ml.

Response of Retinopathy Features

Figure 15-6 compares the progression of microaneurysms and hemorrhages in the two groups over the years. The numbers in the top row indicate the number of eyes which could be assessed at each time interval. The second row indicates the level of significance. The difference between the two groups is significant at all times after the initial assessment. This is not because the control group deteriorated—the mean grading of the eyes which remained assessable changed

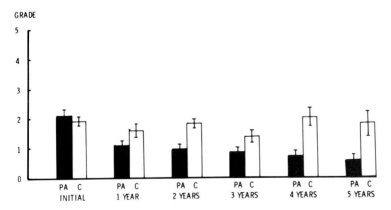

Fig. 15-6. Mean grading plus or minus standard error (SE) of hemorrhages and microaneurysms in the randomly selected pituitary-ablated (PA) and control (C) patients at the different time intervals. P value refers to the significance of the difference between the two.

very little. Rather, it is because of the marked improvement in the pituitary-ablated group, which continues throughout the period of study. Although micro-aneurysms and hemorrhages by themselves are not important as far as visual prognosis is concerned, the improvement is of importance because it indicates an improvement in microvascular lesions.

Hard exudates were not influenced by pituitary ablation, and there was no significant difference between treated and control patients at any time.

Figure 15-7 compares the initial grading of new vessels in the pituitary-ablated group and the control group with the gradings at the different time intervals. The pituitary ablated patients showed an improvement in comparison with their initial assessment at all times. Although the control patients show only slight deterioration, their deterioration, in fact, is best illustrated by the numbers in the top row of the figure, which indicate the number of eyes with new vessels assessed at any particular time in comparison with the number of eyes which had new vessels. For example, at 3 years only 8 out of a total of 23 eyes could be assessed of the control eyes. The other 15 were unassessable because of vitreous hemorr-hage, change to retinitis proliferans, or retinal detachment. All these mean a deterioration or undesirable complication of the new vessels.

Patients with new vessels on the disc have a particularly poor prognosis for vision, and it is this particular feature which shows the improvement most markedly

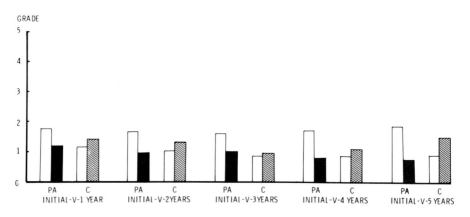

Fig. 15-7. Change in grading of new vessels in pituitary-ablated (PA, *black column*) and control (C, *hatched column*) patients at the different time intervals com-pared with their own pretreatment grading (*clear column*). The fractions above each column indicate the number of eyes which were graded (assessable) out of the total seen at that time with new vessels. P value refers to the difference in the initial and yearly grading of each category.

in those patients who had the operation—provided it resulted in complete ablation. In such patients it is not uncommon to see some degree of optic atrophy.

Visual Acuity

As far as the patient is concerned, the only fact that matters is the effect of the operation on visual acuity. When considering the visual acuity in the better eye (Fig. 15-8) it appears that there is no difference between treated and untreated eyes during the first 2 years. Thereafter the difference becomes greater, and gradually significant levels and almost three lines of difference are reached. From the third year onwards the number of eyes with good vision is higher in the treated group, while the number with impaired vision (20/60 to 20/200) and blind ($<20/200$) is greater in the control group.

New vessels on the disc carry a particularly poor prognosis for vision [4] when untreated. This was not known in 1964, so there was no deliberate randomization for this. However, when the eyes with new vessels on the disc were analyzed in these patients, the difference between treated and control patients was shown already at 1 year when the difference was one and a half lines. This increased to three lines by 4 years and nearly six lines in the few patients studied at 6 years.

There are two further points which need emphasizing. The first one is that in the control group there are 3 patients who had photocoagulation. Photocoagulation was allowed after 1967 if a bleeding point in an "only eye" could be identified, once it produced a vitreous hemorrhage. Such photocoagulation would be expected to destroy new vessels, so that these patients can hardly be regarded as "untreated." Two of these patients maintained vision following phototcoagulation. Although it is not known what the visual acuity of these 3 patients would have been, their inclusion clearly weights the control group favorably.

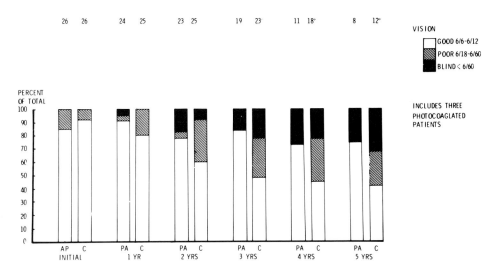

Fig. 15-8. Histograms indicating number of patients with good vision (*clear column*), poor vision (*hatched column*), and blind (*black column*) as percentage of total at the different time intervals in the randomly selected PA and C patients. *Asterisk* (*) indicates 3 photocoagulated patients.

The second point which is not apparent from Figure 15-8 is that while some pituitary implanted patients have lost sight, this has not occurred provided the ablation of the pituitary gland was complete at the first operation. Of the 4 patients who became blind in the pituitary-ablated group, the degree of ablation was only slight in 2 patients, while the other 2 had a second operation after initial ablation. Clearly the second operation was performed too late.

SUMMARY

This controlled randomized study of pituitary ablation showed that the operation arrests or even causes regression of new vessels, microaneurysms and hemorrhages.

In the control patients new vessels advanced and their complications of vitreous hemorrhages and retinitis proliferans were more common than in the treated patients.

The mean visual acuity remained good in pituitary-ablated patients at all times, but deteriorated to poor vision by 3 years in the control patients.

Four of the pituitary implanted patients and 10 of the control patients became blind.

Because of the mortality associated with pituitary ablation and because of the availability of photocoagulation, pituitary ablation is now reserved for patients with new vessels on the disc. For this particular abnormality no other treatment has been proved to be equally effective to the present date.

ACKNOWLEDGMENTS

I would like to thank the many co-workers who helped in this work, in particular Professor Russell Fraser, Dr. G. F. Joplin, and Mr. H. Cheng.

REFERENCES

1. Krieger DT, Sirota DK, Lieberman T: Cryohypophysectomy for diabetic retinopathy: ophthalmological and endocrine correlation. Ann Intern Med 72:309–316, 1970
2. Oakley N, Hill DW, Joplin GF, Kohner EM, Fraser TR: Diabetic retinopathy: I. The assessment of severity and progress by comparison with a set of standard fundus photographs. Diabetologia 3:402–405, 1967
3. Deckert T, Simonsen SE, Poulsen JE: Prognosis of proliferative retinopathy juvenile diabetics. Diabetes 16:728–733, 1967
4. Kohner EM, Panisset A, Cheng H, Fraser TR: Diabetic retinopathy: New vessels arising from the optic disc. I. Grading system and natural history. Diabetes 20:816–823, 1971

Matthew D. Davis

Chapter 16

An Approach To Evaluation of Treatment in Diabetic Retinopathy

I think it is clear that we all share one common goal—that is, to keep our patients seeing as well as possible, for as long as possible, with minimum disruption of their lives by the treatment process itself or by unwanted side-effects of treatment. Outstanding experienced clinicians have somewhat contradictory views on the best available way to achieve this goal. How are we to judge between the various methods of treatment and decide when one or another of them should be applied to any given patient? I submit that there is really only one satisfactory way to approach this problem and that is to conduct a well-controlled study in which various methods are compared with one another and with no treatment. Such a study has been designed, and I might say it has taken a long time, but it is finally initiated. Clearly the most difficult problem in clinical research is the preservation of scientific objectivity while simultaneously giving scrupulous attention to the best interests of each individual patient. I believe that the study which I am presenting will achieve both of these goals.

First of all, we propose in 16 centers across the country to select patients with proliferative diabetic retinopathy or severe nonproliferative retinopathy who still have 20/100 or better vision in both eyes. We then propose, after exhaustive and comprehensive explanation to the patient, to randomly assign one eye of each patient to treatment and the other eye to no treatment (at least temporarily). We then propose to choose, again at random, one of three * treatment techniques for the eye to be treated.

We propose to monitor visual acuity as the single most important variable, but we also propose to carefully document the degree of retinopathy with stereo photographs and to make comparisons within limited groups of patients with very similar retinopathy.

Finally, and I think most importantly, we propose to use what we learn as best we can and as soon as we can to benefit patients in the study. Let us think of what might happen. Our goal is to get 1600 to 1800 patients enrolled in this

---

* Since this presentation the number of treatment groups has been reduced from three to two, eliminating the combined group.

study within a 2-year period. Let us suppose that at the end of 2 or 3 years, when we compare those patients who had surface new vessels not involving the disc and who had these treated with xenon arc photocoagulation, that we find that this particular subgroup has done significantly better than the untreated eyes, and perhaps even significantly better than the eyes treated with argon. We would then propose, when and if that is proven, to look through the current data on all of the untreated eyes of all the other patients; and anyone who has an eye that is in a stage where we have clearly demonstrated that treatment is helpful, will have treatment offered. To withhold treatment at that point would be ethically unjustifiable. I am sure that in this study there are going to be a lot of patients who are blind in both eyes before we get any answers. But I believe the study is ethically justifiable in view of the fact that, at the moment, we do not have any answers.

What are the three treatment techniques? One is argon laser photocoagulation; for brevity, it is essentially what Dr. Little, Dr. Patz, and others are doing—focal treatment plus peripheral scatter treatment. The second type of treatment is exclusively xenon arc and represents a compromise between what a lot of people are doing, namely, focal treatment to new surface vessels and scatter treatment in the periphery. The third treatment technique includes xenon treatment to new surface vessels, much as Dr. Okun and many others have been doing; then a waiting period; and then, if new vessels on the disc or elevated new vessels (fronds in the vitreous) progress, argon treatment is applied to these structures.

At the beginning, photographs are taken of the patient's eyes and are classified. This classification looks at more separate parameters than the Hammersmith classification, but it does not look at any one of them in as great detail; in other words, there are not as many stages; there are not five grades of retinopathy in this classification—there are usually three, although for some parameters there are more.* This is the Airlie House classification published in the book edited by Dr. Morton Goldberg and Dr. Fine, but it has been slightly modified. The first parameter to be graded is hemorrhages and/or microaneuryms. Figure 16-1 is the original Airlie House standard which divides grade 1 from grade 2 in this classification. If there are no red spots at all in the photo being graded, it is rated zero; if there are red spots less than the standard, it is grade 1; and if there are red spots equal to or greater than the standard, it is grade 2. Because there is a long way from nothing to this standard, for this study an additional standard (Fig. 16-2) has been inserted so that we divide this grade into 1a and 1b. The same discussion applies to hard exudates. Figure 16-3 is the original standard and Figure 16-4 is an additional one to divide grade 1 into 1a and 1b. Figure 16-5 has some soft exudates and is used to divide grade 1 soft exudates from grade 2. Figure 16-6 is for venous beading, and it is the original standard in the Airlie House publication. It divides grade 1 venous changes from grade 2. Figure 16-7 is used for two things: new vessels away from the disc and arteriolar abnormalities. As the inferior temporal arteriole disappears under the new vessels it becomes narrow and sheathed. Then it opens up again and has some branches that look like white threads. All of these things are bunched together; the reader

---

* Since this presentation, additional steps have been made in the classification so that now there are five for most lesions. Several additional standard photographs have been added

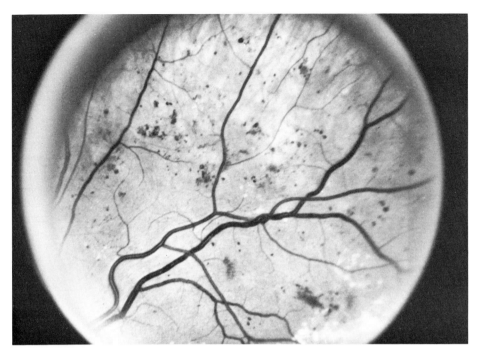

Fig. 16-1. The standard for hemorrhages and microaneurysms; grade 1b has less, grade 2 has same or more (cf. Fig. 16-2).

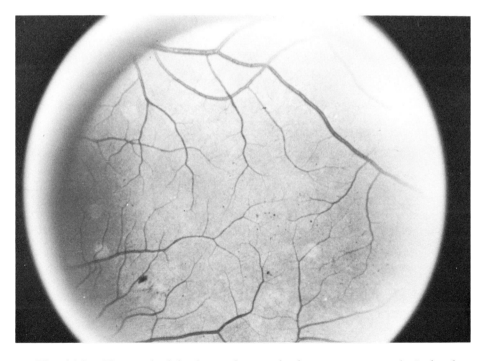

Fig. 16-2. The standard for hemorrhage and microaneurysms; grade 1a has less, grade 1b has same or more (cf. Fig. 16-1).

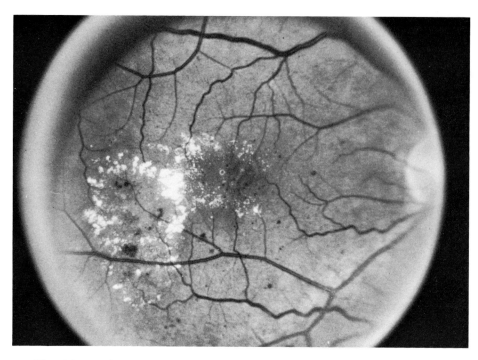

Fig. 16-3. The standard for hard exudates; grade 1b has less, grade 2 has same or more (cf. Fig. 16-4).

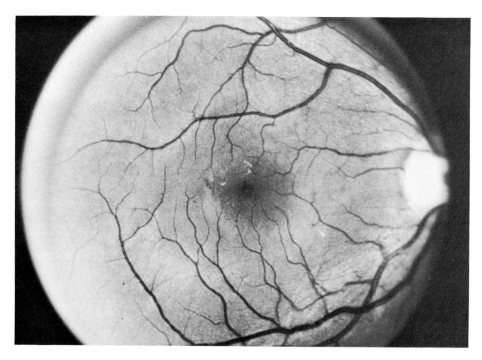

Fig. 16-4. The standard for hard exudates; grade 1a has less, grade 1b has same or more (cf. Fig. 16-3).

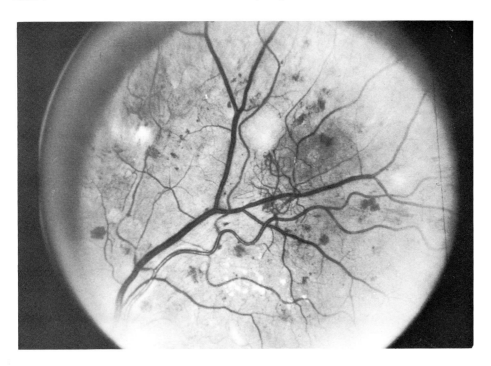

Fig. 16-5. The standard for soft exudates; grade 1 has less, grade 2 has same or more.

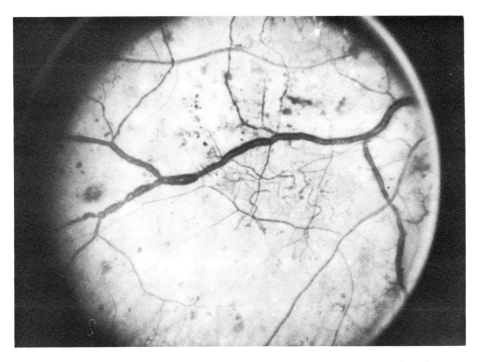

Fig. 16-6. The standard for venous beading; grade 1 has less, grade 2 has same or more.

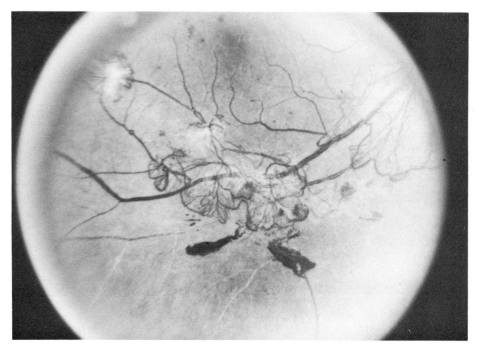

Fig. 16-7. The standard for arteriolar abnormalities and new vessels away from the disc; grade 1 has less, grade 2 has same or more.

makes an eyeball guess as to whether the arterial changes in the field to be graded are as bad as this or worse, or less than this. We also have problems on the other end—the low side—deciding whether there are any changes at all. Figure 16-8 is the standard for intraretinal microvascular abnormalities (IRMAs); this divides grade 1 from grade 2. Figures 16-9 and 16-10 for preretinal hemorrhage; we really do not need two—they were in the original classification just to be sure that someone else using the classification would not ignore the type of preretinal hemorrhage in Figure 16-9 and only grade those with a fluid level. There is about the same amount of hemorrhage in each standard.

We have changed the grading of new vessels a bit; in the current study, new vessels on the disc less than Figure 16-11 are grade 1. As much or more than Figure 16-11 is grade 2, but we have divided grade 2 into 2a, which is less than Figure 16-12 and 2b, which is as bad as or worse than Figure 16-12. These are new vessels on the disc; we consider anything within 1 disc diameter of the disc as being on the disc. Figure 16-13 is the standard for fibrous proliferation on the disc, and Figure 16-14 the standard for fibrous proliferation elsewhere, away from the disc. Figure 16-15, seen in stereo, shows retinal elevation to the left of center and a little bit inferiorly. This is the standard for retinal elevation. The reason for selecting that term is that it is very difficult, as Dr. Okun said yesterday, to know whether you are looking at retinoschisis or retinal detachment, particularly when you are looking at a stereo photograph with nothing else to go on. I must say that even when I have every possible method of examination, I frequently have difficulty telling one from the other in diabetic retinopathy.

We are taking seven standard photographic fields (Fig. 16-16). The first

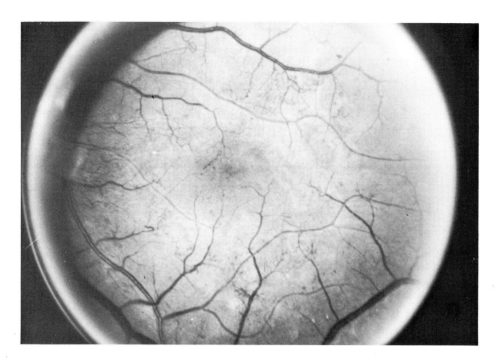

Fig. 16-8. The standard for intraretinal microvascular abnormalities (IRMA's); grade 1 has less, grade 2 has same or more.

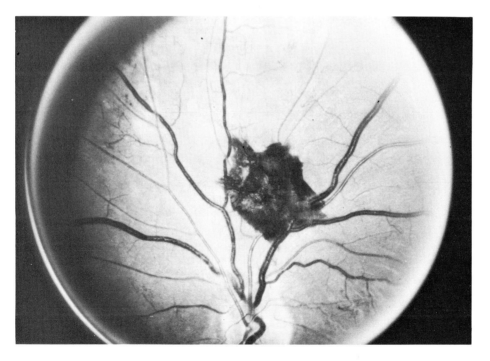

Fig. 16-9. The standard for preretinal hemorrhage; grade 1 has less, grade 2 has same or more (cf. Fig. 16-10).

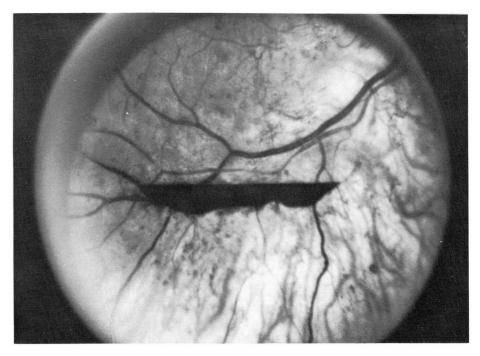

Fig 16-10. Another standard for preretinal hemorrhages with fluid levels; grade 1 has less, grade 2 has same or more (cf. Fig. 16-9).

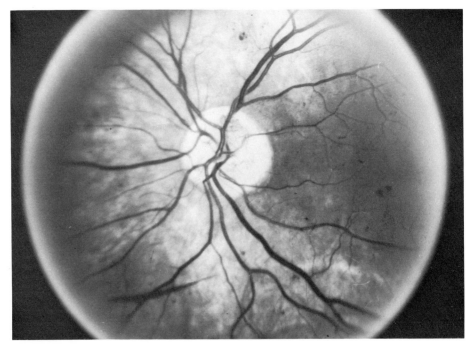

Fig. 16-11. The standard for new vessels on the disc; grade 1 has less, grade 2a has same or more (cf. Fig. 16-12).

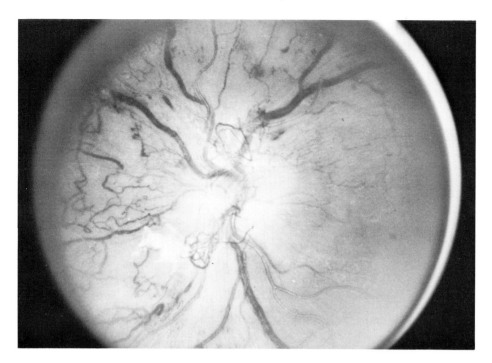

Fig. 16-12.   The standard for new vessels on the disc; grade 2a has less, grade 2b has same or more (cf. Fig. 16-11).

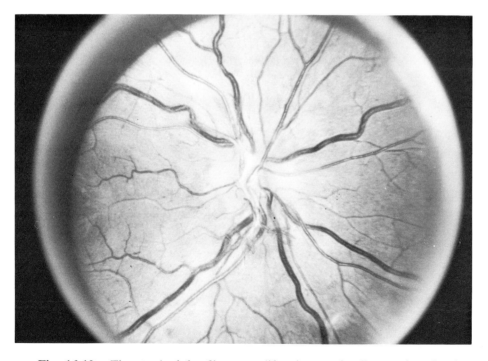

Fig. 16-13.   The standard for fibrous proliferation on the disc; grade 1 has less, grade 2 has same or more.

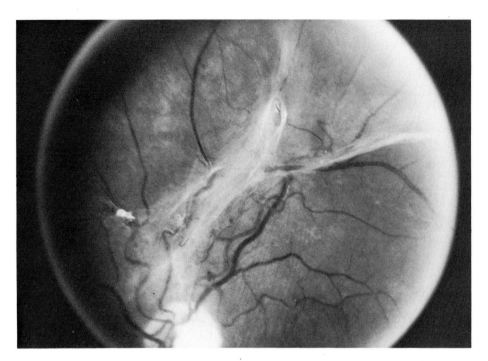

Fig. 16-14. The standard for fibrous proliferation away from the disc; grade 1 has less, grade 2 has same or more.

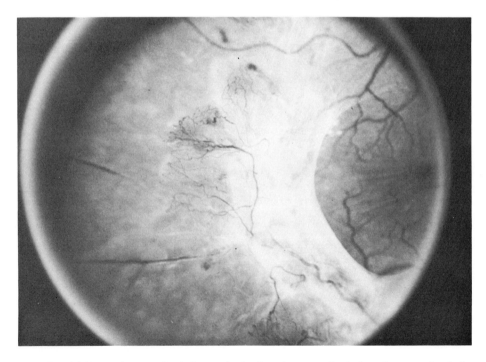

Fig. 16-15. The standard for retinal elevation; grade 1 has less, grade 2 has same or more.

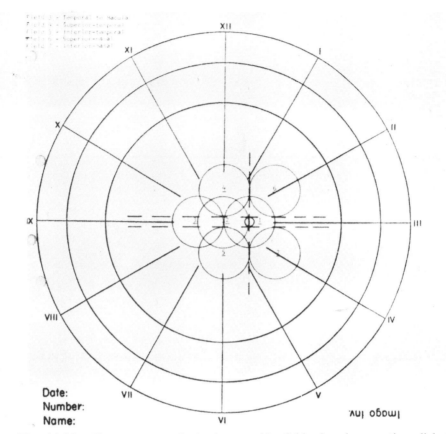

Fig. 16-16. The seven standard photographic fields for documenting diabetic retinopathy.

field is centered on the disc, the second field on the macula, and the third field is temporal to the macula. The remaining four are in the superior temporal, inferior temporal, superior nasal, and inferior nasal quadrants. All are tangent to a vertical line passing through the center of the disc. The superior fields (numbers 4 and 6) are tangent to a horizontal line passing through the upper pole of the disc and the lower fields (numbers 5 and 7) tangent to a horizontal line passing through the lower pole of the disc.

To be suitable for this clinical trial the patient must have proliferative or severe nonproliferative retinopathy. Figures 16-7, 16-11 and 16-12 are examples of proliferative retinopathy that would qualify a patient for entry. Figure 16-17 is an example of what we define as "severe" nonproliferative retinopathy. To qualify for entry, there must be IRMA, venous beading, and soft exudates in any two of the four nonoverlaping standards fields (4, 5, 6, and 7).*

---

* The presence of two out of three of these lesions is sufficient if hemorrhages and/or microaneursysms equal to or greater than Figure 16-2 are present in three of the four non-overlapping fields, plus hemorrhages and/or microaneurysms equal to or greater than Figure 16-18 in the fourth.

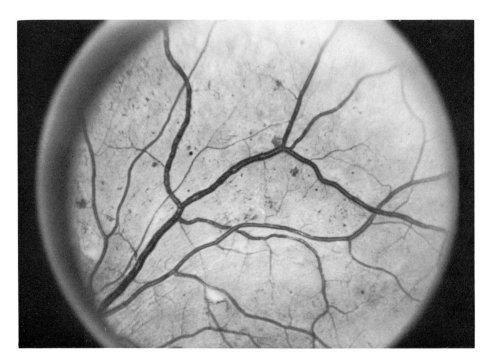

Fig. 16-17. An example of severe nonproliferative retinopathy which has IRMA's, venous beading and soft exudates in any two of the four quadrantic fields.

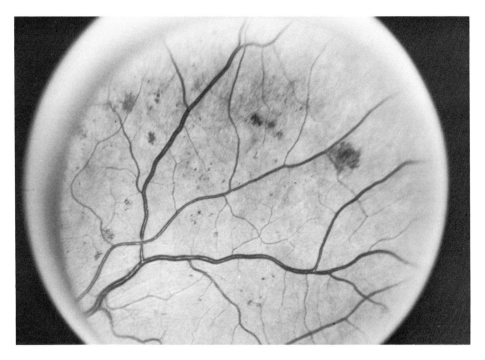

Fig. 16-18. Another standard for hemorrhages and microaneurysms in one or more quadrants, constituting severe nonproliferative retinopathy when accompanied by two of the following: IRMA, venous beading or soft exudates.

Lemuel T. Moorman

Chapter 17
Photocoagulation of the Leaking Diabetic Macula

Diabetes mellitus has been known for many years to cause retinal edema and residual exudate throughout the posterior regions of the eye. The area temporal to the macula has a notable predisposition to edema which is known to be due to abnormally permeable microaneurysms. The spread of this edema into the foveal area has resulted in a significant decrease in central vision in many diabetics who have little or no proliferative retinopathy, and a great deal of useful vision has been lost in these cases in the past without the internist or the ophthalmologist realizing that it is a condition treatable by photocoagulation. Dr. G. Meyer-Schwickerath has been treating this condition since 1955.[1] The first reference to it in the American literature was from several authors quoted in the Proceedings of the Airlie House Conference in 1968.[2-4]

Initially, the treatment consisted of treating the patches of yellow exudate or treating a horseshoe-shaped pattern around the temporal end of the macula. It is now known that the focal treatment of specific clusters of leaking microaneurysms with the argon laser is the effective method of eliminating the macular edema. This was first dealt with in a paper restricted to this subject in 1971.[5] The edema absorbs within 4 to 6 weeks, and there is a concomitant improvement in visual acuity in most cases. Since this type of focal macular leakage is rarely associated with florid proliferative retinopathy, prognosis for prolonged useful vision is much better than the usual case of diabetic retinopathy. The natural course of this condition is that only a few of them resolve spontaneously. When they do, it is over an extended period of time, usually without recovery of useful central vision.

The indications for treatment in this series of 76 eyes has been either the existence of symptomatic macular edema or the presence of a formidable amount of paramacular edema which appeared to be encroaching upon the fovea. Almost without exception, the areas of edema corresponded to specific clusters of microaneurysms which could be observed on fluorescein angiography to have marked leaking of fluorescein dye into the retina. There were a few cases which had so much widespread leaking that a general attack on the microaneurysms had to be made. However, cases of marked generalized retinal leaking without prominent microaneurysms associated with marked edema of the extremities were eliminated on the basis that they were mainly medical problems, or were held over for later evaluation after the peripheral edema was under control with diuretics.

Some of these patients showed a significant increase in central acuity within 1 or 2 weeks following active diuretic therapy. Because of these few cases in which the retinal edema and visual acuity improved on medical therapy, criticism has been made that this is purely a medical condition and should not be treated with laser coagulation. In my opinion, this is not a valid criticism. The cases which respond to the specific treatment of microaneurysms are so clear-cut— usually without any change in the medical therapy—that there is no doubt as to the validity of the treatment of diabetic macular edema in appropriate cases.

Extremely favorable cases are those of short duration (3 to 6 months) with temporal paramacular microaneurysms which can be safely treated with laser coagulation. However, careful treatment in the papillo-macular area can be done with the argon laser with small spot sizes without significantly reducing the central vision. Factors adversely affecting the results (Table 17-1) are associated surface neovascularization in the posterior pole (Figs. 17-1 and 17-2), massive intraretinal vascularization and edema (Fig. 17-3), microhemorrhages within the foveal area (Fig. 17-4), the presence of hard yellow exudates directly in the fovea (Fig. 17-5), marked venous tortuosity, beading and congestion, and lack of perfusion of the macula on fluorescein angiography.

General factors of importance which may adversely affect the treatment are marked diastolic hypertension, severe peripheral edema, and uremia. Control of the diabetes has not been established as an important factor governing the successful treatment of macular edema.

The following cases are presented for interest and illustration of important points:

Case 1. A 57-year-old female diabetic was seen in October 1968, 13 years after the onset of diabetes, with 6/200 vision in the right eye and 20/20 in the left eye. After 3 years of reduced vision, the right macula contained hard exudates and very little residual edema (Fig. 17-6). The left eye showed scattered micro-aneurysms and a few leaking areas in the paramacular area, but no appreciable macular edema (Fig. 17-7). In April 1969 visual acuity in the normal left eye decreased to 20/60 due to the spread of the small amount of preexisting para-macular edema into the fovea. At this time, fluorescein angiography revealed several patches of fluorescein leakage in the temporal paramacular area (Fig. 17-8).

Table 17-1
Factors Adversely Affecting Results

---

1. Surface neovascularization in the posterior pole
2. Massive intraretinal vascularization and edema.
3. Microhemorrhages within the foveal area.
4. Hard yellow exudates directly in the fovea.
5. Marked venous tortuosity and beading.
6. Lack of perfusion of the macula.

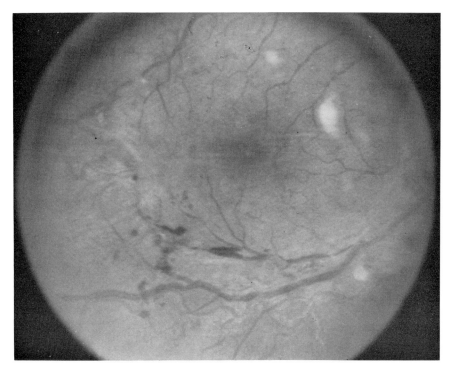

Fig. 17-1. Surface neovascularization in the posterior pole (cf. Fig. 17-2).

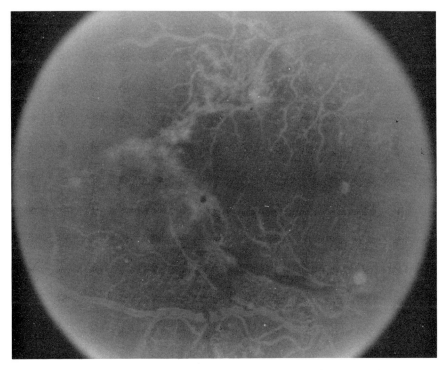

Fig. 17-2. Angiogram of neovascularization (cf. Fig. 17-1).

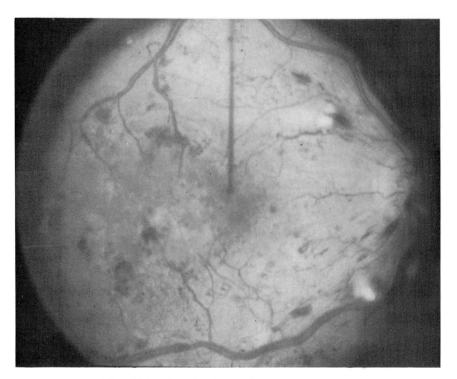

Fig. 17-3. Massive intraretinal vascularization.

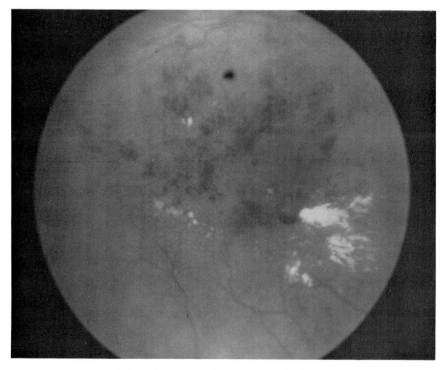

Fig. 17-4. Microhemorrhages in fovea.

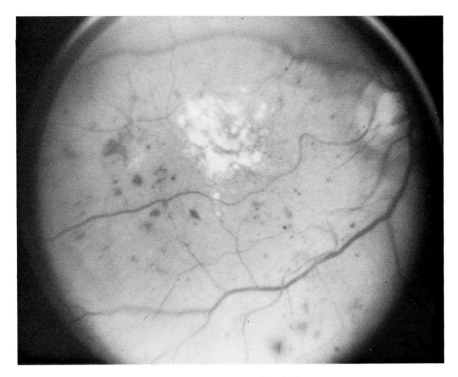

Fig. 17-5. Hard exudate in fovea.

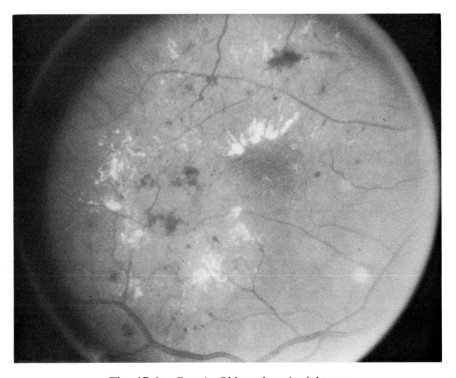

Fig. 17-6. Case 1. Old exudates in right eye.

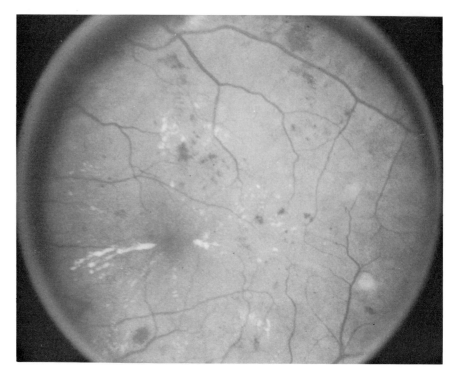

Fig. 17-7. Case 1. Exudative maculopathy; left eye; recent.

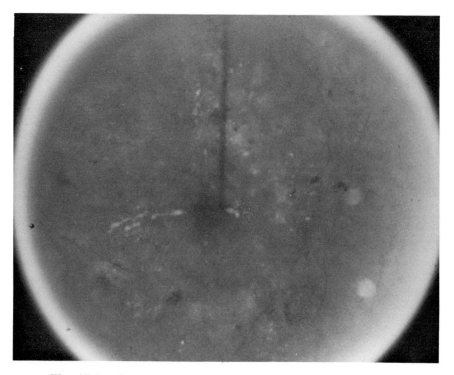

Fig. 17-8. Case 1. Focal leaking in fluorescein angiogram; left eye.

These areas were treated with xenon arc photocoagulation. The visual acuity was reduced to 10/200 by the increase in edema incident to the treatment, but within a month returned to 20/25. When the patient was seen again in January 1970, vision in the left eye was 20/20 and there was no macular edema. The macular area was normal except for occasional microhemorrhages and scattered, photocoagulation pigment scars (Fig. 17-9). The patient was asymptomatic and not aware of any paracentral scotomas.

Comment. This case represents a patient who had lost the vision in the right eye, with a significant resolution of the macular edema without return of vision. The left eye, which was followed until trouble with the edema ensued, was treated successfully with photocoagulation and restored to normal vision. The patient continues to have a normal acuity at the present time.

Case 2. A 73-year-old female diabetic of 9 years' duration had an insidious onset of decreased vision in the left eye for at least several months. When first examined, her visual acuity was 20/40 not corrected with pinhole or lenses. The findings in the fundus were those of circinate exudates upper temporal from the fovea with edema extending into the fovea causing the decreased vision (Fig. 17-10). Fluorescein angiography revealed staining in the clumps of microaneurysms within the circinate area (Fig. 17-11). Argon laser photocoagulation with 50-μ spot size was given May 27, 1971, in multiple areas in which the aneurysms were found (Fig. 17-12). By the time the patient was seen 9 months later, her visual acuity had increased to 20/25 and the macular edema and exudates disappeared. Final photographs show complete clearing of edema and exudates (Fig. 17-13).

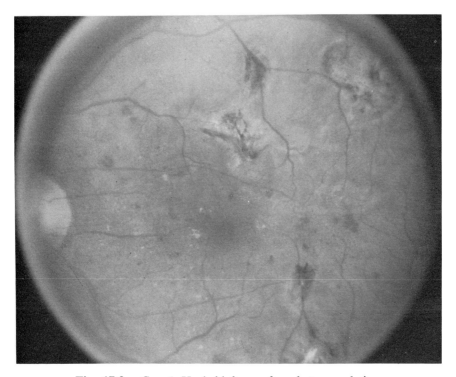

Fig. 17-9.   Case 1. Healed left eye after photocoagulation.

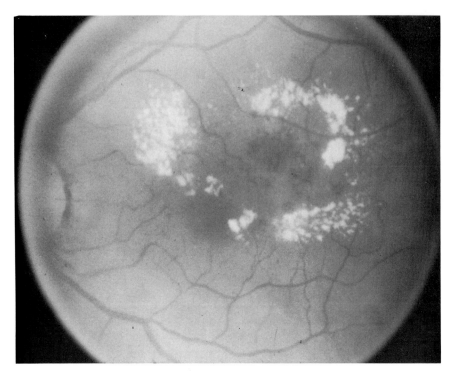

Fig. 17-10. Case 2. Circinate maculopathy with edema.

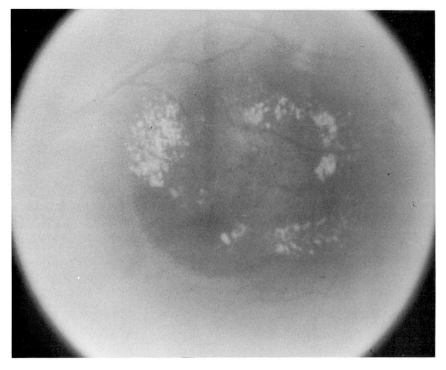

Fig. 17-11. Case 2. Fluorescein leaking from microaneurysms.

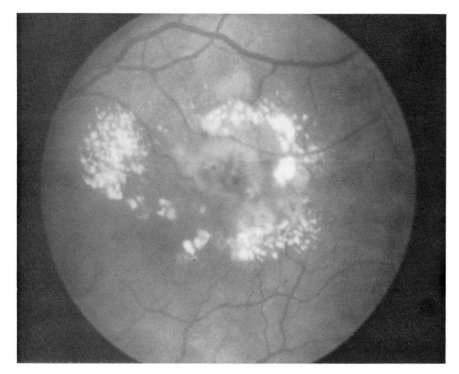

Fig. 17-12. Case 2. Laser treatment of microaneurysms.

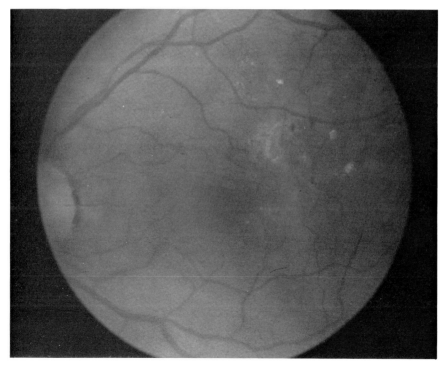

Fig. 17-13. Case 2. Healing after argon treatment; minimal scar.

The patient noticed great improvement in reading and was very happy with the visual result.

Case 3. A 62-year-old female with diabetes of several years duration was being treated on oral insulin. The patient had noticed her visual acuity decreasing for the past 2 to 3 years. About a year previously she was told that there was no treatment. The patient then showed a visual acuity of 7/200 in each eye not corrected with lenses or pinhole. She had marked macular edema with clusters of microaneurysms in both maculae and circinate retinopathy paramacularly (Figs. 17-14 and 17-15). The patient was treated with argon laser photocoagulation in each eye on August 30, 1971, October 8, 1971, and February 29, 1972. Exudates and edema gradually subsided after microaneurysms were destroyed with argon laser. By June 1972 the patient had a visual acuity of 20/80 in the right eye and 20/60 in the left eye with best correction (Figs. 17-16 and 17-17). The patient is extremely happy with her results in that she can now read with a slightly increased add in her bifocal.

DISCUSSION OF RESULTS

The 76 eyes which were treated with either xenon or argon photocoagulation between 1964 and 1972 have a follow-up of more than 6 months (Table 17-2). Of the 76 eyes, 59 were either improved or maintained at a visual acuity of 20/60 or better. Three became worse. Of the 76 eyes, 14 stayed at a relatively stable level, but with a visual acuity of less than 20/60. The eyes which were benefitted

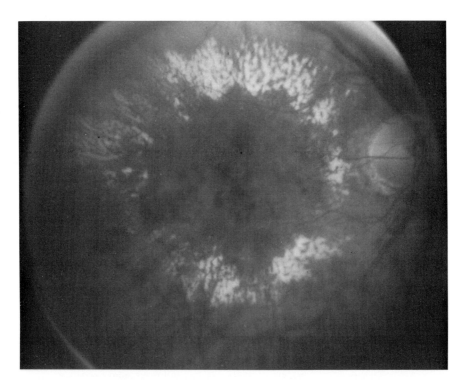

Fig. 17-14. Case 3. Circinate maculopathy; right eye.

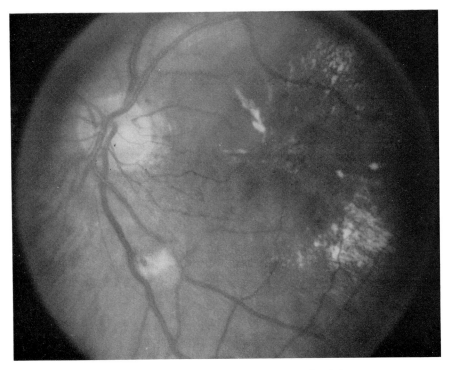

Fig. 17-15. Case 3. Circinate maculopathy; left eye.

did so by virtue of the elimination of foveal edema, but only in rare cases was the edema of the posterior pole completely eliminated.

CONCLUSIONS

Whereas diabetic macular edema is due to a metabolic abnormality of unknown nature, the focal treatment of the microaneurysms which lead to the edema appears to be on a sound footing and the results are significantly better than those in the treatment of proliferative retinopathy. Useful reading acuity can be salvaged in about 3 out of 4 cases.

Table 17-2
Results of Photocoagulation of Leaking
Maculas (6-month follow-up)

Total number of eyes	76
Eyes stabilized at 20/60 or better	59 (77%)
Eyes becoming worse	3
Eyes stabilized below 20/60	14

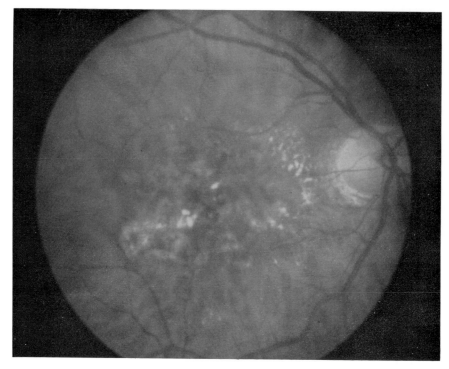

Fig. 17-16. Case 3. Disappearing exudate after argon laser treatment; right eye.

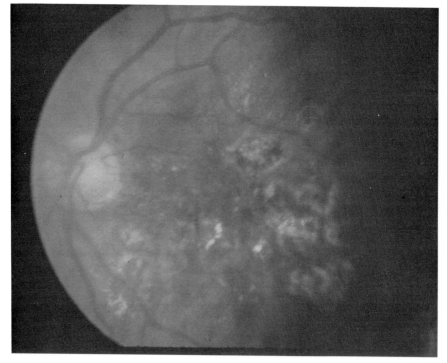

Fig. 17-17. Case 3. Disappearing exudate after argon laser treatment; left eye.

REFERENCES

1. Meyer-Schwickerath G: Personal communication.
2. Wetzig PC, Jepson CN: A review of 232 patients including 401 eyes with diabetic retinopathy. In Goldberg MF, Fine SL (eds): Symposium on the Treatment of Diabetic Retinopathy. US Public Health Service Publ 1890, Washington, 1969, pp 593–601
3. Welch RB: The treatment of diabetic retinopathy. In Goldberg MF, Fine SL (eds): Symposium on the Treatment of Diabetic Retinopathy. US Public Health Services Publ 1890, Washington, 1969, pp 563–567
4. Cleasby CW: Photocoagulation therapy of diabetic retinopathy. In Goldberg FM, Fine SL (eds): Symposium on the Treatment of Diabetic Retinopathy. US Public Health Service Publ 1890, Washington, 1969, pp 465–477
5. Moorman LT, Kenny GS: Photocoagulation of the diabetic leaking macula. Trans Pac Coast OtoOphthalmol Soc 52: 73, 1971

Arnall Patz

Chapter 18
Photocoagulation of Diabetic Disc Neovascularization

Blindness from diabetic retinopathy has increased significantly during the past decade to become the largest cause of new adult blindness in the United States. Many authorities predict that due to the increasing longevity of patients with diabetes, the incidence of diabetic retinopathy will continue to increase strikingly. For example, Field and Kanarek,[1] in a study prepared by the Harvard School of Public Health, indicate that 154,700 persons are now legally blind from diabetic retinopathy and estimate that 573,500 will be blind or visually impaired by the year 2000. Proliferative retinopathy is the usual cause of *severe* visual impairment; and neovascularization emanating from the disc, with its high incidence of vitreal hemorrhage and secondary complications, is a major factor causing visual loss in these patients. Deckert and Paulsen [2] observed that 50 percent of patients with disc neovascularization were blind in approximately 2 years, compared with 5 years for 50 percent of the patients who became blind due to peripheral proliferative retinopathy. A comparison of the natural history of disc versus peripheral proliferative retinopathy in our own series shows an even poorer visual prognosis for the disc neovascularization cases.[3]

The argon laser, which was first introduced by L'Esperance in 1968,[4] provided for the first time an opportunity to treat disc neovascularization directly. The argon laser's high absorption by hemoglobin, high-power density in the focused beam, and precise focusing characteristics permit treatment directly to disc neovascularization.[5,6] Now that the argon laser has become commercially available it is appropriate to present a critical evaluation of its value in the treatment of these patients with diabetic disc neovascularization.

The published reports of others and our own initial observations suggested that, indeed, an effective treatment was now available in these desperate disc neovascularization cases.[7] A critical evaluation of patients followed in a randomized

These studies were supported by a Career Award of The Seeing Eye, Inc., Morristown, New Jersey, and a grant from the National Eye Institute, National Institutes of Health, Bethesda, Maryland.

controlled study showed that the long-term observations were much less favorable than initially observed in our own patients. Indeed, one group of patients receiving only a single treatment to the disc neovascularization fared poorer in the treated eye than in the untreated control. In the course of the treatment of approximately 250 consecutive disc neovascularization patients, a technique has been developed that, at least in our hands, led to more successful obliteration of the vessels with significantly fewer complications from treatment. These methods are presented in this report.

TREATMENT TECHNIQUE

The management of diabetic disc neovascularization cases can be conveniently divided into three sections:

1. The identification of afferent or feeder vessels to the neovascularization by fluorescein angiography;
2. Application of the minimal amount of energy necessary to occlude neovascularization and repeating treatment when vessels reopen in order to minimize risk of damage to the optic nerve and the nerve fibre layer of the adjacent retina, and to reduce the complication of hemorrhage;
3. Ablation of the retina posterior to the equator, sparing the papillomacular zone.

Identification of Feeder Vessels

The intravenous injection of 5 cc of 10-percent fluorescein by standard technique is performed and the angiogram is recorded on TRI-X film. The power supply to the fluorescein camera unit should ideally permit photographs to be taken at the rate of at least one frame per second. The camera should be equipped with the Allen stereo separator or comparable device to permit stereo photographs. The TRI-X negatives should be examined directly with a stereo viewer to obtain best resolution of the feeder vessels.

It is desirable in the actual treatment to have available a stereo negative and positive set of transparencies of the early transit phase. A convenient method of viewing is to attach a standard stereo viewer above the eye pieces of the slit-lamp viewing oculars (Fig. 18-1A). Other aids in identification which are helpful but not as useful as the stereo viewer are the projection of a negative or positive transparency onto a screen behind the patient or by the use of a simple TV camera and monitor to enlarge the negative. The TV camera-monitor device permits instant switching from negative to positive viewing; but this, as well as the projection system, lacks the added resolution that can be obtained in the stereoscopic viewing of the negative. Also, an 8 by 10 enlargement of the feeder vessel can be attached to the slit lamp for reference. Recently, in collaboration with Robert Flower of the Applied Physics Laboratory of Johns Hopkins University, a special viewer has been constructed which enables the superimposition of the standard color fundus photograph with a positive black-and-white transparency of the fluorescein angiogram in the early transit phase. Feeder vessels seen with fluorescein angiography can be conveniently extrapolated to the slit-lamp view of the fundus during treatment Fig. 18-1B. We are at present testing this superimposition device in the treatment of patients with disc neovascularization. The

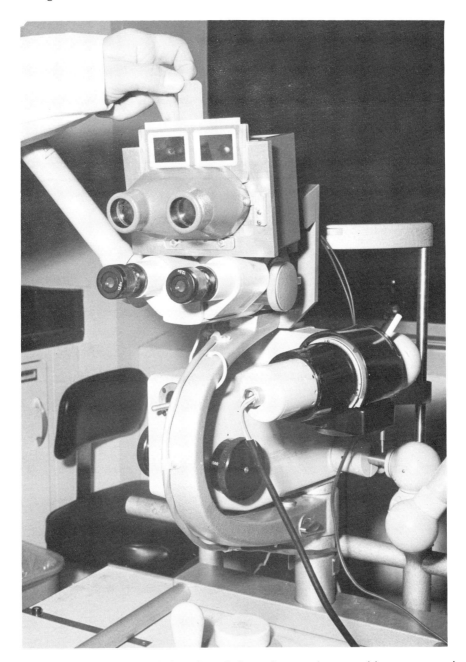

Fig. 18-1A. Stereoscopic illuminated viewer for negative or positive transparencies of the fluorescein angiogram shown mounted above the oculars of the slit lamp of the laser photocoagulator.

simple stereo fluorescein viewer, shown in Figure 18-1A, appears to be the most practical and simple in our preliminary evaluation of these different devices.

Using the stereoscopic viewing of negatives and positive transparencies, we have been successful in identifying feeder vessels to the disc neovascularization in

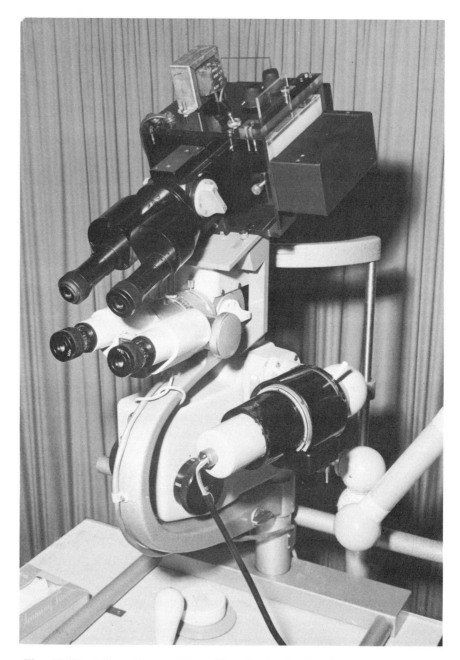

Fig. 18-1B. Viewer for superimposition of color fundus photograph and fluorescein angiographic picture. The device permits rapid extrapolation of the fluorescein land-marks to the color photograph.

approximately 40 percent of the cases. The actual technique described below is based on the management of those patients where a feeder vessel(s) is identified. A slight modification of this technique is subsequently described which has proven useful in some of those remaining cases where a definite feeder pattern cannot be established.

A slit-lamp delivery system utilizing either the low-vacuum contact lens or the Goldmann posterior fundus lens is required to obtain the best stereoscopic resolution of the vascular components of the frond. For most cases, a retrobulbar anesthetic is not required. However, when there is the least instability of fixation or lack of cooperation, a retrobulbar injection is routinely administered.

The patient is placed at the slit lamp with the stereo fluorescein positive transparency or negative placed in the viewer immediately above the eye pieces. The fluorescein pattern is extrapolated to the stereo slit-lamp view through the contact lens.

Minimal Application of Energy and Repetition of Treatment

Although there is apparently minimal absorption of the argon energy by the nonpigmented nerve tissue of the optic disc, an unknown amount of heat is probably transferred from the blood in the vessels of the frond that are not elevated. Also, the treatment requires application of laser energy to the peripheral part of the disc frond which usually overlies the retina with its underlying pigment epithelium. For these two reasons, minimal application of laser energy is recommended.

To avoid excess energy application to the frond, determination of the baseline power for photocoagulation of the eye under treatment is first performed. Since the physical transmission of the argon laser beam will vary according to the transparency of the media, it is convenient to establish the milliwattage power required to obtain a moderate intensity retinal burn in the pigment epithelium. This can be placed near the disc inferior or nasal to the disc margin utilizing the 50-μ spot size setting. This serves as a power reference point to start treatment over the disc.

TREATMENT OF FEEDER VESSELS

Utilizing the 50-μ spot size and 0.1-second time exposure, power is applied starting at about one-half the baseline power reading. The power is gradually increased until some fragmentation of the blood column, or narrowing of the feeder vessel, is observed. At this point the blood flow will be appreciably reduced in the frond, but some blood flow will be present and blood will still be present in the more peripheral parts of the neovascularization.

TREATMENT OF PERIPHERY OF THE FROND

After this preliminary treatment of the feeder vessel, the spot size is increased to 200 μ unless the periphery of the vascular network overlies the major retinal branch vessels, when it may be preferable to use the 100-μ spot-size setting. It is important to specifically avoid utilizing the 50-μ spot-size setting at this point because, in our experience, the high-power density here will frequently produce hemorrhage when treating the peripheral part of the frond. The power setting is gradually increased until significant slowing, or stopping, of the blood flow is noted with fragmentation of the blood column throughout the frond. At this point in the treatment the 50-μ spot-size setting may be used cautiously in the peripheral components of the frond, if necessary, to treat adjacent to the major retinal vessels. When treating over the periphery of the frond, it is desirable to increase the duration of photocoagulation to 0.2 seconds and specifically avoiding very short pulses of energy at 0.05 seconds, or shorter.

Treatment is then directed to other lesions in the fundus, if present. These include microaneurysms, shunt vessels (intraretinal microvascular abnormalities), surface or elevated neovascularization away from the disc, and small red dots that are either hemorrhages or microaneurysms. In addition, the scatter or so-called "ablation" photocoagulations, which are described below, are started. The disc neovascularization is then reexamined. Since the original changes may have been due partly to spasm, some of the vessels will have partially reopened while treating in the periphery; further treatment on the disc is repeated as originally described.

The patient should be reexamined later the same day or on the following day. In most cases, some of the previously closed vessels will have reopened, and additional treatment is applied to these vessels as described above. Particular care should be made to start with a one-half baseline power setting using a spot size setting of 200 μ, and no smaller than 100 μ when treating the periphery of the disc frond as the blood flow is usually appreciably reduced and the energy more efficiently absorbed at re-treatment. The 50-μ spot-size setting should be carefully avoided unless one is re-treating a very narrow lumen feeder vessel. The patient should then be reexamined in 24 to 48 hours, at which time some of the vessels will probably have reopened and the treatment should be repeated as just described. We have found that at least two—and more frequently three or four separate treatment sittings—are required to achieve satisfactory closure of the vessels and fragmentation of the blood column in the vascular frond; however, in occasional patients the treatment has been repeated as many as five times within the first week of the initial treatment.

Re-treatment over the peripapillary retina can be done with reasonable safety *only* during the first few days after the *initial* treatment while the retina is still edematous and thickened. In 6 to 10 days the retinal edema and thickening subsides and increased pigmentation gradually occurs along with atrophy of the outer retinal layers.

The patient should be returned for examination in approximately 3 weeks to determine if residual vessels are present and if new vessels have developed. It is extremely important that this examination be made at this time so that further treatment, as needed, can be done before significant new vessel proliferation has occurred. The same procedure is utilized as before; however, no longer can treatment be applied over the peripapillary retina without risk of nerve fiber layer damage due to thinning of the previously treated retina and the presence of proliferated pigment epithelium. It is not necessary generally to repeat the fluorescein study at this first return series of treatments. Here, again, the treatment of the disc vessels is divided into from one to three separate sittings as just described. If any areas of peripheral ablation treatment are found inadequate, the additional treatment to the peripheral retina is performed to cover the area posterior to the equator and, in addition, if any peripheral diabetic lesions are noted they are also treated.

The patient is then returned in approximately 3 to 4 weeks for reevaluation and, again, patent vessels of the frond are re-treated. A final evaluation is made approximately 1 month later. Then the patient is examined regularly at approximately 3-month intervals. No further treatment to the disc new vessels is advocated at this time as the chances of successfully obliterating the frond are considered poor and the risk of hemorrhage at treatment too great to warrant additional treatment.[8]

Retinal Ablation

An examination of the records of our initial disc neovascularization patients treated, with a minimal follow-up of 1 year, reveals that those patients having had simultaneous and extensive treatment of peripheral vascular lesions showed, in general, appreciably better obliteration and less recurrence of the disc new vessels. The extensive peripheral treatment involved large areas of the fundus, photocoagulating all aneurysms, small hemorrhages, intraretinal microvascular abnormalities, and surface neovascularization not involving the papillomacular bundle. These preliminary results are consistent with the published reports of Meyer-Schwickerath[9] and Aiello[10] and the unpublished observations of Little[11] on the value of peripheral ablation in selected cases of disc neovascularization. Indeed, the unpublished observations of Little[11] prompted our retrospective review of disc patients treated by repeated focal treatment with minimal peripheral photocoagulation and those having combined extensive peripheral treatment.

Peripheral ablation is done with the application of between 1000 and 1600 photocoagulations with the 500-μ spot-size setting, or 500 to 800 with the 1000-μ spot size, during the initial treatment series. The ablation pattern is oval in shape, extending to one and one-half disc diameters superior, temporal, and inferior to the fovea, and one disc diameter superior, temporal, and nasal to the disc. When within the temporal arcade of vessels, 200-μ spot-size coagulations are used.

DISCUSSION

Behrendt[12] demonstrated the feasibility of differentiating an afferent flow pattern in selected cases of diabetic neovascularization. Treatment of the afferent or "feeder" vessels of the neovascularization effectively stops the blood flow through the frond temporarily. In only occasional cases this has given permanent obliteration of a part of the neovascular tuft in our hands, and in most patients we have observed that the vessels reopen within approximately 1 week. It is for this reason that we have applied the principle of re-treatment during the first few days after the initial treatment, in order to apply further energy while the blood flow in the neovascularization is still diminished from the original treatment and the retina adjacent to the disc is edematous. The thickened and somewhat opaque retina insulates the pigment epithelium from the additional energy during the repeat treatment sittings. This protective effect is helpful only during the initial series of treatments, as the retina ultimately becomes thinned and the pigment epithelium hypertrophied in the treatment scars. Subsequently re-treatment over the retina adjacent to the disc then carries a significant risk of permanent nerve fiber bundle damage.

In the treatment of our earlier disc neovascularization cases, the frequency of significant hemorrhage was in the 20-percent range. Furthermore, the frequency of recurrence or increase in the proliferation was significant. Indeed, in our controlled study the initial group of treated patients having only one argon laser treatment fared less well in the treated eye than in their untreated "control" eye. A single treatment appeared to stimulate further proliferation more frequently than it helped reduce the severity of the neovascularization.

Multiple repeat treatments on the disc without extensive peripheral treatment or planned ablation type of therapy was found in the controlled study to be only very slightly better than the natural history in the untreated matched control eye. The slight difference was not significant statistically.[13]

The high incidence of hemorrhage in our early cases may have resulted in part because of the ability to focus down to 30-μ spots of coagulation with our original argon laser developed at the Wilmer Institute. Furthermore, there was a tendency to do much heavier treatment in one session because a retrobulbar anesthesia was required with the direct ophthalmoscope delivery system then in use. By changing to the slit-lamp binocular delivery system and avoiding small spot-size settings, and by using much less energy application at individual treatment sessions, a reduction in significant hemorrhages at treatment or within a few days after treatment from 20 percent down to approximately 3 percent has resulted.

When the high-power density of the focused 50-μ spot is applied to larger caliber vessels in the frond, especially when they are on the efferent side of the neovascularization, a hemorrhage can occur from rupture of the vessel wall without complete coagulation through the width of the lumen. As a general rule, the coagulating beam should always be at least one and one-half times the diameter of the vessel lumen being treated. Most of the disc hemorrhages that have occurred in our more recent cases resulted from the 50-μ spot-size settings on the peripheral portions of the frond with larger caliber vessels, and the use of short-pulsed applications of energy at 0.05 seconds, or occasionally 0.1 seconds. By treating feeder vessels initially to slow down the vascular flow, then treating the remainder of the frond with larger spot-size settings of 200 μ, and always no smaller than 100 μ for 0.2 seconds or longer the incidence of hemorrhage at or shortly after treatment has decreased significantly.

When a hemorrhage occurs at treatment, the spot-size setting should be increased immediately, and photocoagulation applied to the blood overlying the bleeding site. The energy is increased until the hemorrhage stops. In addition, the intraocular pressure can be raised by pressing the low-vacuum or Goldmann contact lens firmly against the globe.

When no feeder pattern to the disc neovascularization can be identified, a slight modification of the treatment plan has been adopted. Frequently, but not always, the vessels that are slightly narrower in caliber are on the afferent side of vascular flow in the frond. Starting with 100-μ spot-size settings, energy is gradually increased while treating these smaller vessels on the disc until fragmentation of the blood column or significant narrowing of the vessel results. The periphery of the frond is then treated with 200-μ or not smaller than 100-μ spot-size settings, as already described.

When the fluorescein angiogram provides no clue to the vascular flow characteristics of the frond, or if the patient cannot have fluorescein injection, the following technique has been utilized for focal treatment of the disc vessels. The baseline power to get a threshold lesion beneath the disc is determined. The spot-size setting is adjusted to 200 μ and the power setting adjusted to one-half the threshold power reading. Using a minimum time exposure of 0.2 seconds with a 200-μ spot-size setting, treatment is gently applied to the peripheral components of the disc new vessels. The energy is gradually increased until fragmentation of the blood column results. Particular care is given to avoid overtreatment by turning the blood column to a char black color. Diabetic lesions peripheral to the disc vessels are then treated in the same manner as described under "feeder vessel technique." While the patient is still seated at the slit lamp, at the completion of the peripheral treatment, the disc vessels are reexamined. Generally, most of the previously fragmented blood columns in the disc frond will have demonstrated a return of blood flow, and re-treatment is done using 200-μ spot-size coagulations and occasionally 100-μ spot-size when treating immediately adjacent to the underlying retinal vessels.

SUMMARY AND CONCLUSIONS

The major cause of severe visual loss in patients with diabetic retinopathy has been the complications of disc neovascularization. Attempts to obliterate disc neovascularization produced a significant number of complications in our earlier treatments attempts. In addition, a single photocoagulation was found to carry a poorer prognosis than occurred in the untreated control eye.

By the use of the feeder vessel technique and the application of multiple treatments, avoiding excess energy and small spot-size photocoagulations on the periphery of the frond, a significant reduction in hemorrhages resulted and more effective vessel obliteration was achieved.

Careful examination of the patients—hourly after treatment—showed that many of the vessels had reopened within a few hours, and within 4 to 7 days 40 to 75 percent of the previously closed neovascularization would have become patent. These observations led to the divided treatment schedule. The apparent better results on treated disc neovascularization cases when extensive peripheral retinal photocoagulation was performed simultaneously, together with the results of other investigators, suggest that peripheral retinal ablation may be a useful adjunct in the management of disc neovascularization. Preliminary observations in patients followed up to 20 months with focal treatment on the disc, combined with peripheral ablation, are consistent with this observation.

The duration of follow-up and the number of cases treated with this divided schedule of treatments and peripheral ablation are still insufficient to establish conclusively that the treatment is definitely beneficial. Further controlled studies in a larger number of patients with longer follow-up will be required to document the true role of photocoagulationn treatment for diabetic patients with neovascularization emanating from the optic disc.

REFERENCES

1. Field R, Kanarek P: Diabetic Retinopathy and Blindness; Presented at the Annual Meeting of the National Society for the Prevention of Blindness, New York City, 1972

2. Deckert T, Simonsen SE, Poulsen JE: Prognosis of proliferative retinopathy in juvenile diabetics. Diabetes, 16:728–733, 1967

3. Patz A, Berkow JW: Visual and systemic prognosis in diabetic retinopathy.

Trans Amer Acad Ophthalmol Otolaryngol 72:253–257, 1968

4. L'Esperance FA Jr: An ophthalmic argon laser photocoagulation system: Design, construction, and laboratory investigations. Trans Am Ophthalmol Soc 66: 827–904, 1968

5. Zweng HC, Little HL, Peabody RR: Laser Photocoagulation and Retinal Angiography. St. Louis, Mosby, 1969

6. Patz, A, Schatz H, Ryan SJ, Berkow JW, Lazarus, MG: Argon laser photocoagu-

lation for treatment of advanced diabetic retinopathy. Trans Am Acad Ophthalmol and Otolaryngol 76:984–989, July-August 1972

7. Patz A, Maumenee AE, Ryan SJ: Argon laser photocoagulation—advantages and limitations. Trans Am Acad Ophthalmol and Otolaryngol 75:569–577, May-June 1971

8. Patz A: A guide to argon laser photocoagulation. Surv Ophthalmol 16:249–257, 1972

9. Meyer-Schwickerath G: Light Coagulation. St. Louis, Mosby, 1960

10. Beetham WP, Aiello L, Balodimos MC, Koncz L: Ruby laser photocoagulation of early diabetic neovascular retinopathy. Arch Ophthalmol 83:261–272, 1970

11. Little HL: personal communication

12. Behrendt T: Argon laser coagulation. Arch. Ophthalmol, 1970

13. Patz, A: Photocoagulation Therapy of Diabetic Disc Neovascularization (to be published)

Arnall Patz

Chapter 19

Adjuncts to Photocoagulation Therapy
of Diabetic Maculopathy

In patients with maturity-onset diabetes, background diabetic retinopathy with macular involvement was the largest cause of visual impairment in our Diabetic Center. In patients with juvenile-onset diabetes and florid proliferative retinopathy, approximately 20 percent demonstrated significant macular edema at some time during their follow-up. Many of these patients with longer standing macular edema developed varying degrees of cystoid maculopathy.

The macular edema in the juvenile-onset diabetic frequently underwent spontaneous regression to a significant degree when the patients were followed over a period of a few years. On the other hand, patients with adult-onset diabetes showing macular edema rarely showed spontaneous regression and generally showed gradual deterioration when followed over a period of several years. Patients with maculopathy of adult-onset diabetes frequently showed a reasonable degree of symmetry in the two eyes and lent themselves well to a randomized controlled study of photocoagulation treatment for one year.[1]

Because of the major concern for the proliferative component of the retinopathy, the associated macular edema in these cases has not been infrequently overlooked, or at least its effect on central visual acuity not fully appreciated. In contrast, in adult-onset diabetes the macular edema more often occurred in background retinopathy or in those cases with only minimal proliferative changes.

A controlled study on the role of argon laser photocoagulation in adult-onset diabetic maculopathy has been presented in detail elsewhere. In summary, the study included patients with visual impairment to 20/40 or poorer. The eye selected for treatment was assigned on a random basis. The follow-up in these patients has been from a minimum of 9 months up to a maximum of 3 years following treatment. Patients were recruited from June 1969 through December 1971, and followed until September 1972 at which time the data were evaluated.

These studies were supported by a Career Award of The Seeing Eye, Inc., Morristown, New Jersey, and a grant from the National Eye Institute, National Institutes of Health, Bethesda, Maryland.

251

The response in the treated eye was shown to be significantly better than in the untreated eye. Therapy was rated successful if visual acuity either improved or remained stable while the other eye continued to deteriorate. In occasional instances of maculopathy the treated eye fared poorer than the untreated eye. From January 1, 1972 to the present time the majority of patients with adult-onset diabetes showing background diabetic retinopathy with macular edema had both eyes treated by argon laser photocoagulation.

ADJUNCTS TO THERAPY

Several adjuncts to therapy were found useful in planning and performing treatment in these cases with diabetic maculopathy:

1. Standard stereo color photography was used to document the degree of macular edema.
2. Multiple fixation Polaroid photographs were used to establish precisely the fixation point and stability of fixation. It was important to obtain the fixation photographs prior to regular fundus photography and especially prior to performing fluorescein angiography to avoid the photic stress on the macula from these repeated flash exposures.
3. Extrapolation of the high contrast fluorescein photographic details to the fundus view were obtained through the slit lamp and contact lens. Several methods were evolved, culminating in a special viewing device. These methods in their order of development were as follows:

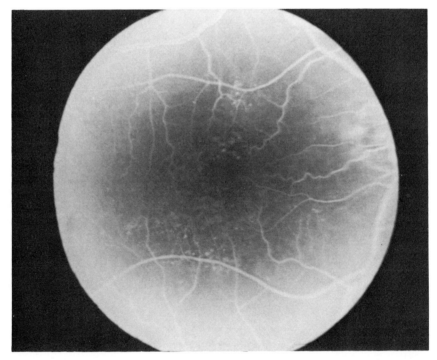

Fig. 19-1A. Early retinal transit phase of fluorescein angiogram from a 58-year old diabetic female with a known history of diabetes for 16 years. Multiple microaneurysms and intraretinal microvascular abnormalities are noted in the perimacular area (cf. Figs. 19-1B and 19-1C).

a. Placing an 8-by-10 positive print enlargement of a selected fluorescein angiography frame adjacent to the patient;

b. Projection on a screen behind and above the patient of a 2-by-2 negative or positive fluorescein transparency;

c. Use of a TV camera and monitor to enlarge the fluorescein negative to either positive or negative mode on a 12-by-14 TV monitor screen;

d. Inserting stereo negatives or positive transparencies in a specially illuminated viewer clamped above the stereo eye pieces of the laser slit lamp, (Fig. 18-1*A*).

e. Development of a special beam splitter viewing device with separate illumination to a color fundus photograph and fluorescein transparency. Superimposition of the separate images to give precise orientation of fluorescein leakage points to the color photographic landmarks and hence the fundus contact lens landmarks (Fig. 18-1*B*).

Fluorescein angiograms were studied in reference to (1) areas of nonperfusion of the retinal capillaries, (2) aneurysms, (3) shunt vessels, and (4) the degree of dye leakage (Fig. 19-1). It was significant that in occasional cases bright red dots seen on ophthalmoscopy and color photography and thought to be isolated microaneurysms did not fill or stain with fluorescein. Presumably, these were hyalinized aneurysms with red blood cells trapped in the lumen. In several cases large aneurysms would light up brightly in the early fluorescein transit but showed no significant leakage in the late phases. On the other hand, shunt vessels and

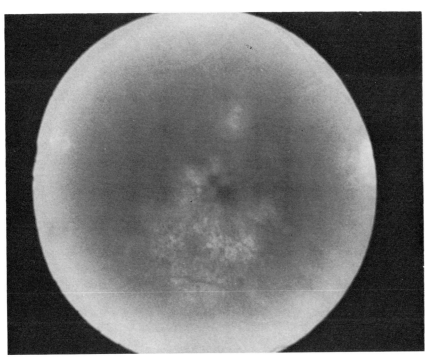

Fig. 19-1B. Four minutes after photograph shown in Figure 19-1A shows marked leakage extending into the center of the macula. Visual acuity is reduced in this patient to 20/20 (cf. Fig. 19-1C).

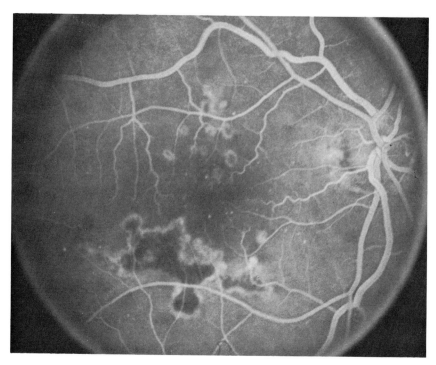

Fig. 19-1C. One year following argon laser photocoagulation. Visual acuity has improved to 20/30. An occasional microaneurysm is noted in the macular area.

aneurysms in areas of retinal edema could only be hazily visualized in either the color photographs or by ophthalmoscopy, but in the fluorescein photographs they frequently showed significant dye leakage, particularly in later phases of the dye transit. These observations have clinical significance and indicate that the bright red spots visualized during treatment about the macula should not necessarily be treated unless fluorescein studies have demonstrated definite leakage qualities. This is especially important in the papillomacular bundle area where minimal treatment is advocated.

Although our controlled study on the photocoagulation treatment of the maculopathy of adult-onset diabetes showed the treated eye to fare significantly better than the untreated control, there was much to be desired in the ultimate therapeutic results. It is important to point out that successful treatment in the majority of patients meant holding onto visual acuity at the level prior to treatment whereas the untreated eye continued to deteriorate, or that the rate of deterioration in the treated eye was slower than that in the untreated control. Only a small percentage of the treated eyes actually showed significant improvement. Further research studies are indicated toward improving photocoagulation methods and also directed towards the prevention of capillary nonperfusion about the macula and the other parameters of the maculopathy.

Although fluorescein angiography performed prior to treatment furnishes more precise landmarks for placement of the photocoagulation, it is not yet proven that this added precision gives a better therapeutic result than the random treatment of "red spots" and other obvious vascular lesions seen grossly.

Our recent studies [2] on fluorescein capillary perfusion patterns about the macula are useful in predicting the natural history of diabetic macular edema and also the response to photocoagulation therapy. Patients showing poor perfusion in the central macula area, with the border of the perifoveal vascular net occluded, showed an unfavorable prognosis. On the other hand, patients with normal capillary perfusion in the immediate area of the macula demonstrated a good prognosis following photocoagulation treatment with the following exceptions. Patients showing severe hypertension or renal decompensation invariably fared poorly with photocoagulation treatment, even when capillary perfusion was normal in the macular area; also, patients with good central perfusion but with advanced cystoid maculopathy responded poorly. Patients with early cystoid changes generally responded favorably.

SUMMARY AND CONCLUSIONS

Fluorescein angiography is a useful adjunct in treatment of patients with diabetic maculopathy when it is desirable to precisely locate the areas of capillary and other microvascular abnormalities. The actual contribution of the fluorescein studies to the ultimate therapeutic results will require further documentation.

When using fluorescein photographic data during treatment, it is important to provide a rapid and convenient method to extrapolate the high-resolution fluorescein photographic details to the view of the fundus seen through the slit lamp and contact lens. The utilization of an 8-by-10 enlargement placed adjacent to the patient, a stereo viewer placed over the eyepieces of the slit lamp, a projector imaging the enlarged photograph on a screen behind the patient, the use of a TV camera and monitor screen to image the negative, and the use of a superimposition viewer for color and fluorescein photographs have been used. The simple stereo viewer attached to the top of the oculars of the slit lamp has proven most useful in our experience and the instrument is simple to operate and inexpensive to construct.

REFERENCES

1. Patz A, Schatz H, Berkow JW, Gittelsohn AM, Ticho U: Macular edema—an overlooked complication of diabetic retinopathy. Trans Am Acad Ophthalmol Otolaryngol 77:34, 1973

2. Ticho U, Patz A: The management of macular edema in patients with diabetic retinopathy. Am J Ophtholmol, 76:880, 1973

Marvin D. Siperstein

Chapter 20
Electron Microscopic Diagnosis of Diabetic Microangiopathy

Dr. J. S. Friedenwald was clearly the first to suggest that thickening of capillary basement membranes represents the underlying lesion of diabetic vascular disease in the eye and in the kidney.[1, 2] With this pioneering observation, many investigators have asked the question: Is the microangiopathy that is observed throughout the body of the diabetic characterized by a similar thickening of the capillary basement membrane; and if so, can this lesion be quantitated objectively and reproducibly so that the relationship of diabetic microangiopathy to the other variables of diabetes—control, age, onset of hyperglycemia—could be studied?

The problem that faced the investigator in this field was clearly, first, how to obtain tissue that could be studied in life and, second, how objectively to quantitate capillary basement membrane width. Various investigators attacked the problem looking at either skin or muscle capillaries—the two tissues readily susceptible to biopsy. The initial studies from our laboratory,[3] from Paul Lacy's laboratory at St. Louis,[4] from Schwartz's laboratory in Chicago,[5] and from the University of Pittsburgh,[6] all made use of skin capillaries. The problem involved in quantitating capillary basement membrane width in the skin is shown schematically in Figure 20-1. Unfortunately, for the aim of these studies, the basement membrane of skin capillaries is normally laminated, fragmented, and hence very difficult to quantitate. As a result, each of the three investigating groups, including ourselves, after publishing rather equivocal studies, abandoned the use of skin biopsies.

Several groups of investigators then turned to the study of muscle capillaries, initially obtained only at surgery.[7-11] The schematic diagram in Figure 20-1 also illustrates that muscle capillaries, in contrast to skin, possess a basement membrane that is fairly homogenous and readily quantitated. The results of these earlier

From the Department of Internal Medicine, The University of Texas Southwestern Medical School at Dallas, Dallas, Texas. Current address is the Department of Medicine, University of California Service, Veterans Administration Hospital, San Francisco, California 94121. This work was supported by USPHS AM 13866; Dr. Siperstein was the recipient of Research Career Award HE 1958.

CAPILLARY BASEMENT MEMBRANES

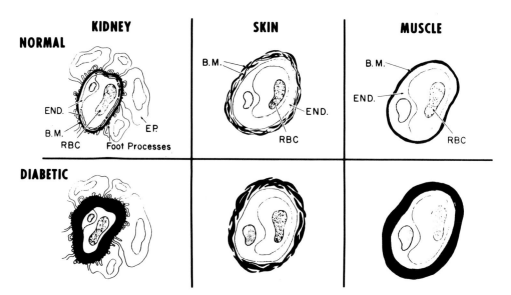

Fig. 20-1. Schematic drawings of normal and diabetic capillaries in three frequently biopsied tissues.

studies were not uniform but they were certainly suggestive. Zachs et al.[7] were the first to use electron microscopic measurements. We do not know from what site the muscle was obtained, nor did they indicate their method. Only 4 patients were studied, but 3 of the 4 diabetics were said to show thickened basement membranes. Bloodworth[10] published on only 2 diabetic patients, but both of those showed thickening. A rather subjective approach by Bencosme *et al.*[8] indicated 12 of 16 diabetic patients had thickened basement membranes, and Fuchs[9] used abdominal muscle and found 3 of 3 thickened. So, what I am about to describe really represents a modest conceptual extension of what these four investigators have already indicated: namely, that capillary basement membrane thickening probably is a hallmark of diabetes mellitus. But, clearly, with these very small numbers of samples one could not state such a conclusion with any statistical confidence.

What was needed then, as I have already anticipated, was a means of obtaining such tissue in life without resorting to open biopsies or the collection of tissue at the operating table. Our laboratory therefore simply modified the Franklin–Silverman needle to use it to biopsy the quadriceps muscle, consistently obtained at a point halfway between the knee and the thigh.[11] This general technique with a few modifications has been adopted by all subsequent investigators. The technique of measuring the basement membrane is extremely simple and quite reproducible; we simply photograph 15 capillaries randomly and overlay a grid of 20 radiating lines; wherever the lines cross the basement membrane, it is measured at right angles to a tangent to the endothelial cell. One can analyze such data statistically with a high degree of confidence. The technique is clearly laborious in that one makes 20 measurements of each capillary, and, as a result, there have been several attempts to simplify this procedure suggested in the literature. On theoretical grounds, Williamson et al.[12] have suggested that it would be better and simpler to measure only the two narrowest sites on the basement membrane. The theoretical objection to this approach is that basement membrane thickening tends to be focal; hence, if one looks at a diabetic capillary there are areas where the basement membrane is grossly thickened and other areas where it is thin. If one now ignores those areas where it is thick and looks only at the two thinnest areas of basement membrane, the degree of diabetic microangiopathy should be grossly underestimated. And, in part as a result of this selectivity, Williamson's method has proved to be a relatively insensitive means of detecting microangiopathy.

The first question to be asked when employing an objective technique and statistically significant numbers of capillary basement membrane measurements is simply: Is capillary basement membrane thickening a consistent finding in diabetic subjects? It is. Our initial studies, published now some 5 years ago—based on 50 normal subjects and 51 diabetics—indicated a highly significant difference between the normal and the diabetic.[13] We have considerably extended the number of patients, but the average values have not changed significantly. Roughly, a normal capillary basement membrane measured in this way is 1100 Å wide, a diabetic capillary averages 2400 Å, i.e., approximately twice that of the normal. There is a minor error involved in these absolute figures since by the method of measuring that I have just described one will frequently obtain oblique sections through a capillary. The resulting error can be calculated at about 10 to 12 percent.[14] So, by the technique we are employing, to correct these figures to absolute cross-sectional basement membrane width, the numbers should be lowered by this small correction factor.

From the practical standpoint, of course, one wishes to ask the critical question: What is the prevalence of this lesion in a diabetic and a normal population? If a "normal" basement membrane is defined as having a width of less than 1325 Å and "diabetic" at 1600 Å and above, the false-positive error of the method is remarkably small at 1 percent and the sensitivity of this method—namely, 93 percent of diabetics—is remarkably high.[13, 15] The lesion is almost ubiquitous. Data from the deltoid, quadriceps, and gastrocnemius indicate that at each of these sites there is thickening of the basement membrane in the diabetic.[13] There tends, however, to be some increase in the degree of thickening as one moves caudad, the deltoid being thinner than the quadriceps which, in turn, is slightly thinner than the gastrocnemius. This progression is clearly not due to hydrostatic pressure since one can dissociate capillary basement membrane width from hydrostatic pressure in an individual or even in a giraffe.[16] Moreover, the most cephalad tissue we have biopsied—namely, the cerebral cortex—shows almost exactly the same basement membrane width as that in the quadriceps muscle, roughly 1100 Å in the normal, 2200 Å in the diabetic.

The next question that we wish to ask is: If there is a relationship between the carbohydrate abnormalities of diabetes and the degree of microangiopathy, is there a correlation between the thickness of the basement membrane and the duration of the diabetes defined as the duration of hyperglycemia? For the first 10 to 15 years—the range where the data are sufficiently large to be significant—there is clearly no such correlation. One can make two points from these data. First, even at the outset of overt diabetes mellitus, basement membrane thickening in muscle is maximal; secondly, even with longstanding diabetes there is no significant progression of basement membrane width in the muscle capillary. The latter finding is unfortunate from a practical standpoint because it is obvious that in the eye and in the kidney, capillary basement membrane thickening does progress with duration of hyperglycemia, as every clinician knows and as has recently been documented by careful quantitative electron microscopy.[17] The muscle capillary basement membrane technique cannot therefore be used to predict the degree of microangiopathy from one tissue to another. This weakness of the technique appeared for a time to be overcome by Williamson et al.[16, 18, 19] when, in preliminary reports, they reported that by their procedure one could detect a relationship between duration of hyperglycemia and basement membrane width. In fact, from their completely published data [20] it is now clear that they, too, find no durational effect on basement membrane width for at least 10 and probably even for 20 years.

Capillary basement membrane thickening in muscle, therefore, occurs earlier than in kidney, and as a result muscle capillary basement membrane measurements represents a more sensitive means of detecting diabetic microangiopathy. On the other hand, one cannot, at least after the onset of hyperglycemia, relate width of the capillary basement membrane in muscle to that of kidney or eye, and perhaps other tissues where progression of the basement membrane width clearly does occur.

The observation that thickening of capillary basement membrane is usually present at the time of onset of hyperglycemia—noted by us and confirmed by Williamson et al.[20]—suggests that there may be a dissociation between hyperglycemia and the microangiopathic lesion of diabetes mellitus. This finding of course has again raised the question: Is hyperglycemia responsible for diabetic microangiopathy? The data from our group, and we would suggest from Williamson's laboratory, would both strongly suggest that it is not.

Another way of approaching this problem is to determine whether hyperglycemia in animals will produce microangiopathy, i.e., basement membrane thickening, in the absence of genetic diabetes mellitus. Alloxan hyperglycemia has been widely used for this purpose; and I can summarize the literature by stating that no one has produced quantitative data showing thickening of any capillary basement membrane in any tissue following the administration of alloxan. The most careful study to date is that of Bloodworth et al.[21] They looked at the hyperglycemic dog kidney, measured the glomerular basement membrane width, and found that in age-matched groups there is no significant basement membrane thickening. We have done a similar study [22] in the monkey in collaboration with Dr. Gordon E. Gibbs from the University of Nebraska. There is no difference between the muscle capillary basement membrane width in normal and alloxan-treated monkeys even after 4 to 12 years of hyperglycemia.

One can do the same experiment in man. If one looks at secondary hyperglycemia of man, from whatever cause, basement membrane thickening is rarely found. For example, in patients with chronic pancreatitis, with one exception in 18, all have muscle capillary basement membrane widths below 1600 Å. The average is not significantly different from normal. We have studied several other causes of secondary diabetes—hyperlipemia, pheochromocytoma, Cushing's disease, and acromegaly—without finding basement membrane thickening. This observation now has been confirmed by Danowski [23] and more recently by Camerini-Devalos et al.[24]

It follows that one of the practical uses of this approach is in the diagnosis of those individuals who have unequivocal hyperglycemia and in whom one suspects a secondary cause of this chemical abnormality. If one cannot see basement membrane thickening by using the sensitive electron microscopy method, it is unlikely that the patient with hyperglycemia has diabetes mellitus. From a practical standpoint these results suggest that it is very unlikely that hyperglycemia not due to genetic diabetes will produce microangiopathy, either in animals or in man.

The other approach to the question of the relationship between hyperglycemia and microangiopathy is to look at genetically prediabetic subjects, defined in this study as the offspring of two diabetic parents. There are only two secure ways to define genetic prediabetes with any degree of confidence: as the offspring of two diabetic parents or the nondiabetic identical twin of a diabetic. In either case, the ultimate prevalence of overt diabetes is high. If we look at the offspring of two diabetic parents, we should have a large group of individuals in whom we can accurately predict the presence of two diabetic genes. When we do this and then exclude any evidence of carbohydrate abnormality or abnormalities in insulin secretion or growth hormone secretion, we find, using a variance analysis method, that we can detect a 74-percent prevalence of statistically significant microangiopathy.[15] Moreover, this figure has progressively increased over the subsequent years since the initial biopsies. These data, obtained in a prospective manner, would indicate that basement membrane thickening in the patient who is destined to become overtly diabetic consistently precedes the appearance of glucose intolerance.

Taken together, these findings can be summarized as follows: By an objective, relatively simple method of quantitating basement membrane width in muscle, one can demonstrate that diabetic microangiopathy is for practical purposes a *sine qua non* of genetic diabetes, basement membrane thickening being present in between 93 and 98 percent of overtly diabetic subjects. Secondly, this lesion is not found in animals or in man in the absence of genetic diabetes mellitus despite longstanding hyperglycemia in patients with pancreatitis for as long as 13 to 14 years. These facts would suggest that the hyperglycemia of diabetes mellitus is not the cause of the microangiopathy of this disease. This suggestion is strongly supported by the observation that the prediabetic subject—the offspring of two diabetic parents— who carries two diabetic genes but who does not have any detectable glucose abnormality will show diabetic microangiopathy by this technique in at least 74 percent of cases. Taken together, then, these data would suggest that diabetic microangiopathy represents an early, independent, and perhaps even the primary lesion of the diabetic syndrome.

ACKNOWLEDGMENTS

I wish to express my sincere gratitude to Mr. Henry Burns and Ms. Stevonne Gulley for carrying out the electron microscopy and to Mrs. Mary Ellen Plummer for performing the morphometric analyses.

REFERENCES

1. Friedenwald JS: A new approach to some problems of retinal vascular disease. Am J Ophthalmol 32:487, 1949

2. Friedenwald JS: Diabetic retinopathy. Am J Ophthalmol 33:1187, 1950

3. Siperstein MD, Colwell A, Meyer K

(eds): Small Blood Vessel Involvement in Diabetes Mellitus. Washington, DC American Institute of Biological Sciences, 1964, p 125

4. Banson BB, Lacy PE: Diabetic microangiopathy in human toes. With emphasis on the ultrastructural change in dermal capillaries. Am J Pathol 45:41, 1964

5. Friederici HHR, Tucker WR, Schwartz TB: Observations on small blood vessels of skin in the normal and in diabetic patients. Diabetes 15:233, 1966

6. Pardo V, Perez-Stable E, Fisher ER: Electron microscopic study of dermal capillaries in diabetes mellitus. Lab Invest 15:1994, 1966

7. Zacks SI, Peagues JJ, Elliott FA: Interstitial muscle capillaries in patients with diabetes mellitus: A light and electron microscopic study. Metabolism 11:381, 1962

8. Bencosme SA, West RO, Kerr JW, Wilson DL: Diabetic capillary angiopathy in human skeletal muscles. Am J Med 40:67, 1966

9. Fuchs U: Elektronenmikroskopische Untersuchugen menschlicher Muskelcapillaren bei Diabetes mellitus. Frankfurt Z Pathol 73:318, 1964

10. Bloodworth JMB Jr: Diabetic microangiopathy. Diabetes 12:99, 1963

11. Siperstein MD, Norton W, Unger RH, Madison LL: Muscle capillary basement membrane width in normal, diabetic and prediabetic patients. Transactions of the Association of American Physicians, Vol LXXIX, Collingdale, Pa., Dornan, 1966, p 330

12. Williamson JR, Vogler NJ, Kilo C: Estimation of vascular basement membrane thickness. Theoretical and practical considerations. Diabetes 18:567, 1969

13. Siperstein MD, Unger RH, Madison LL: Studies of muscle capillary basement membranes in normal subjects, diabetic and prediabetic patients. J Clin Invest 47:1973, 1968

14. Siperstein MD, Raskin P, Burns H: Electron microscopic quantification of diabetic microangiopathy. Diabetes 22:514, 1973

15. Siperstein MD: Capillary basement membranes in diabetes. In Fajans SS, Sussman KE (eds): Diabetes Mellitus: Diagnosis and Treatment, Vol III. New York, American Diabetes Association, 1971, p 281

16. Williamson JR, Kilo C: Basement membrane thickening and the mystery of diabetes. Hosp Prac 1:109, 1971

17. Hansen R: A quantitative estimate of the peripheral glomerular basement membrane in recent juvenile diabetes. Diabetologia 1:97, 1965

18. Williamson JR, Vogler NJ, Kilo C: Muscle capillary basement membrane changes in diabetes mellitus. Diabetes 19, 356, 1970 (abstr)

19. Williamson JR, Vogler NJ, Kilo C, Daughaday WH: Muscle capillary basement membrane thickening (CBMT) in subjects with mild carbohydrate intolerance. Diabetes 20:329, 1971 (abstr)

20. Kilo C, Vogler NJ, Williamson JR: Muscle capillary basement membrane changes related to aging and to diabetes mellitus. Diabetes 21:881, 1972

21. Bloodworth JMB Jr, Engerman RL, Powers KL: Experimental diabetic microangiopathy. 1. Basement membrane statistics in the dog. Diabetes 18:455, 1969

22. Siperstein MD: The relationship of carbohydrate derangements to the microangiopathy of diabetes. In Cerasi E, Luft R (eds): Pathogenesis of Diabetes Mellitus. Nobel Symposium 13. Stockholm, Almqvist & Wiksell, 1970

23. Danowski TS: Muscle capillary basement membrane in juvenile diabetes mellitus. Metabolism 31:1125, 1972

24. Camerini-Davalos RA et al: Deterioration of tolerance to glucose and progression of the microangiopathy. Diabetes 21:321, 1972 (abstr)

Chapter 21
Panel Discussions

Dr. Davis. I would like to make a couple of comments relative to Dr. Siperstein's presentation (Chapter 20). I think it can be demonstrated that what we ophthalmologists call diabetic retinopathy in trypsin digest preparations can be produced in alloxan diabetic dogs. Dr. Siperstein makes one assumption which I would like to disagree with, and that is that muscle capillary basement membrane thickening more or less equals diabetic microangiopathy. The only way I can explain his findings and our findings is to assume that these are two different things.

It is quite clear that there is something different in the retina of our alloxan diabetic dogs than there is in normal controls of the same age. That does not mean that occasionally one or two aneurysms do not occur in the control dogs in the retinal periphery; they do. But there are no control dogs that have as many—and I am quoting from memory, and I may be a little bit off—as five or six aneurysms in one retina. And there are 14 out of 14 dogs that have been diabetic for more than 4 years that show substantially more retinopathy than this. So, the only conclusion that I can draw is that the muscle capillary basement membrane thickening, which as Dr. Siperstein has shown, doesn't seem to change with duration of diabetes is not the fundamental process underlying retinopathy. We all know that the microangiopathy that we see, and that makes our patients go blind and that kills them, is related to duration; so the only conclusion I can draw is that muscle capillary basement membrane thickening is not as closely related to the microangiopathy we see as Dr. Siperstein suggests.

Dr. Siperstein maintains that if we could demonstrate that the angiopathy in the alloxan diabetic dog was less if he was well controlled and if his blood sugar was better controlled than in another group of dogs whose control was poor, that he would then agree that this was honest-to-God experimentally induced diabetic microangiopathy. That experiment is underway. It has not been going on long enough to get an answer, so we have to leave that question unresolved. But I would like to ask Dr. Siperstein how he feels we should put all this together, assuming that we do demonstrate that alloxan diabetic dogs develop less retinopathy if they are well controlled than if they are poorly controlled. Where do we go from there with our speculation and theorizing?

263

Dr. Siperstein. Dr. Davis' comments imply a number of questions; let me answer the last one first. If in man or in animals one really produced diabetic microangiopathy with hyperglycemia alone, then I am wrong. I repeat: It has never yet been done. The reason I say that is that repeatedly over the years, especially according to Dr. Bloodworth's group, hyperglycemia will produce renal microangiopathy. He has published pictures of lesions in the kidney and said that this was nodular intracapillary glomerulosclerosis. When *objective* measurements of renal basement membrane width were finally published, as I showed you, there was not even basement membrane thickening demonstrable. I think we simply have to see whether the lesions that are being produced are at all specific. In the kidney one can produce basement membrane thickening from all sorts of insults and diseases that are not diabetes mellitus, e.g., nephrosis, lupus, and so on. Complex disease, injecting foreign protein, and injecting alloxan represent a damaging agent to capillaries. It has been well known that alloxan is a general toxic agent, which is why one would like to segregate hyperglycemia per se from the general toxicity of alloxan. It would be nice to show such lesions in the absence of alloxan injection; pancreatectomized animals would be one such model, as man pancreatectomizes himself, in our experience, with alcohol, but does not produce basement membrane thickening by this procedure.

So what I am saying is that the control is a critical one. In the absence of objective data and such control, we have no evidence that hyperglycemia will produce basement membrane thickening.

I do not think I have glossed lightly over the dissociation between duration of hyperglycemia and basement membrane thickening. I emphasized it repeatedly. This is a weakness of the method, but it indicates that basement membrane measurements in muscle represent a more sensitive measure of diabetic microangiopathy, not a less sensitive one. It simply means, as the prediabetic studies demonstrate, that basement membrane thickening in muscle occurs before hyperglycemia. This observation has now been widely confirmed; Frackel, who initially denied the association, has now found a 100-percent frequency of basement membrane thickening; the group in Pitttsburgh under Donowsky has recently confirmed the observation; and Dr. Bloodworth, himself, has just reported that the prediabetic subject, in fact, is characterized by a thickening of muscle capillary basement membrane. I do not think there is any question amongst anyone in this field that muscle capillary basement membrane thickening, in general, is the hallmark of diabetes mellitus. Dr. Friedenwald was absolutely right.

Dr. Davis. I did not mean to say that Dr. Siperstein had glossed over the matter of duration of diabetes and its relation to basement membrane thickening; but why does capillary basement membrane thickening equal diabetic microangiopathy? That is what I do not understand, Dr. Siperstein.

Dr. Siperstein. Because it is regularly associated with genetic diabetes mellitus and no other disease in man or animals, save perhaps lupus.

Dr. Davis. Fine. You have demonstrated to my satisfaction that it is a marker of genetic diabetes. That does not necessarily equate it to the microangiopathy that is seen in the retina and in the kidney. The one thing that every paper about the vascular complications of diabetes agrees upon is that they are related to duration. And now you have a finding that is not related to duration and you want to equate the two things. That seems to me to be at best questionable.

Dr. Siperstein. No, I think there is a logical fallacy there. The lesion is a hallmark of diabetes, its progression in one tissue need not a priori be the same as in any other tissue. That is a general phenomenon in any genetic disorder; not every tissue is similarly affected by any genetic disorder I know. The qualitative lesion is identical; the difference is that the rate of progression is different—it's faster in muscle than in other tissues, up to the point of hyperglycemia at which it plateaus in muscle. I do not think that makes it a separate lesion; it makes it a more rapidly progressive lesion.

Dr. Davis. My contention is that you have not demonstrated that it is not possibly a separate lesion. You said before that if our well-controlled dogs had less retinopathy than poorly controlled dogs that "you were wrong." I think you are going too far there. Your data are there; your data are not wrong. Isn't it just a matter of having to change our interpretation of the data, if there are new data? I personally feel confident that 5 years from now, when we talk, we will be together trying to make all the facts fit, and that will mean the theory will have to be modified but not the facts; the interpretations, not the data.

Dr. Siperstein. All I can say is that Dr. Bloodworth made the same prediction 5 years ago and he has retracted it.

Dr. Kohner. I would like to make two comments. The first one is, I do not think genetic diabetes is the only cause of basement membrane thickening; I believe that Williamson from St. Louis found that acromegalics who admittedly may be prediabetic, but are not genetically diabetic, also had a high proportion of muscle basement membrane thickening.

The second comment is that we are all talking about manifestations of a biochemical abnormality as yet not clearly defined. Dr. Siperstein states that basement membrane thickening is the earliest abnormality he can find. I would like to remind you of the work of Ceresi and Luft reported in 1967. They did glucose infusions into babies of diabetic parents, and as early as 6 weeks after birth the babies demonstrated an abnormality of insulin response.

I think that whether we talk of hyperglycemia or of basement membrane thickening we are talking about a metabolic abnormality which we have not clearly defined because we do not know what it is. I think it is something to do with insulin and these are just manifestations of the abnormality. The question really is, What are we going to treat? Are we going to treat manifestation of this abnormality as seen by high blood sugar, or are we going to try to prevent this manifestation of high blood sugar by keeping the patient thin, to try to prevent factors which we know will bring on diabetes? Or are we going to treat basement membrane? I myself do not know how to treat basement membrane. I know a little bit more about how to control high blood sugar, but I want to emphasize that we are just treating a manifestation of the abnormality and not the basic abnormality itself. But obviously, we cannot treat a basic abnormality until we know what it is.

Dr. Goldberg. In a related question, is there any evidence other than the renal evidence you cited, Dr. Siperstein, that basement membrane thickening has any pathophysiologic effect? In other words, does it cause disease?

Dr. Caird. The situation in the kidney is very different from that in muscle. As far as secondary diabetes goes, Ireland et al. (1967) has shown quite conclusively that basement membrane thickening does occur in the kidney in chronic pancreatitis; there is no doubt about this at all. Secondly, Osterby (1971) has shown conclusively that there is progressive membrane thickening in the kidney after the development of fasting hyperglycemia.

One other point: one's chances of getting diabetes are increased—other than by having diabetic parents—by having a lot of children. Women with more than five children have about five times the chance of developing diabetes than women with no children (Middleton and Caird, 1968). Does Dr. Siperstein note any relationship between basement membrane thickening and parity in his prediabetic retinopathy?

Dr. Zweng. Dr. Siperstein, in your cut-off between normal and diabetic to give a high incidence of predictability, and so on, there was a gap between 1325 and 1600 angstroms. Was there a fair number of subjects that fell into that 275-Å gap?

Dr. Siperstein. The answer is sort of implicit in the data in that the equivocal range obviously only includes subjects that don't fall below or over the two numbers and I think that comes out to 6 or 8 percent, it's very small. So the method is quite useful and the equivocal range is minor. It is not bimodal; I think that is worth emphasizing. I thought that's what you were going to ask and even though you did not, I think that the technique simply is not going to be that good to actually show bimodility; of course, it would be wonderful if you could. But that is going to have to await a far better technique than we devised. Yes, if many causes of hyperglycemia really produce retinopathy, then I think one has a very strong argument for hyperglycemia producing retinopathy. I would have no argument with that. I think retinopathy, as Dr. Goldberg presented it, can be quite non-specific. Numerous toxic stimuli will produce microaneurysms, and I think one would like to see the same experiment performed in man. We have taken repeated retinal photographs of our pancreatitis patients for many many years, as you might expect, since we want to be the first to find these lesions, not the last. And they have not developed microangiopathy, nor have they developed basement membrane thickening.

The problem of whether diabetics have more or less children is still being argued. Steinberg thinks that fertility is increased in diabetics, but very slightly. Whether you can aggravate some underlying genetic predisposition to diabetes by having numerous children, by being overweight, or by various other insults seems very likely. But it does not follow that having five children predictably leads to diabetes mellitus. That is a very different sort of question. We have not studied multiparous patients in terms of basement membrane thickening, but I would not think it would be very fruitful, since most patients who have 10 children never become diabetic. I quoted Ester B. Hanssen. Her data present the most objective demonstration that basement membrane thickening in the kidney precedes and continues after hyperglycemia appears; of course, that is exactly what I am saying. There is a difference between the progression of basement membrane thickening in the kidney and in the muscle. I think I have now said it five or six times.

Yes, Dr. Eirman's study of pancreatitis showed one classic lesion in his nodular intracapillary glomerulosclerosis. The problem of the nonspecific thickening of the basement membrane in the kidney has been commented upon by many people, in addition to myself, and it's a very difficult lesion to pin down. Many things will cause basement membrane thickening in the kidney but not in muscle. So, this is evidence against what I am saying but I would not say it is strong evidence, although there are pathophysiologic implications of basement membrane thickening besides the kidney which is certainly the cause of death; renal failure is the commonest cause of death amongst juvenile diabetics; so that lesion is life-threatening, life-taking. In the nerve there are certainly good data that show that involvement of the basement membrane does impair blood flow or oxygenation. There is certainly implicit data but certainly not convincing data that the vasovasorum may be involved in compromising of oxygenation to the thickened intima of large vessels. But beyond that, I repeat, no one knows. That does not mean that one cannot equate basement membrane thickening with diabetic microangiopathy. It simply means that we do not have the bridge between thickening of the basement membrane and all tissues, and the effects of diabetes which do not affect all tissues, but only some. Muscle does not necrose very regularly in the diabetic despite the basement membrane thickening actually.

The studies of Luft, which I suspect he still does believe, showed that if you infuse a very large dose of glucose into normal people, 20 percent of them will show a depression in the secretion of insulin. In the identical twins of the diabetics, probably all but one has shown this suppression of insulin secretion. That means that if you infuse massive amounts of glucose, you can demonstrate some decrease in insulin with a tremendous error. But that does not mean that insulin deprivation causes diabetic microangiopathy. Practically total insulin deprivation for one or two decades in man—pancreatitis patients—in the absence of genetic diabetes mellitus does not lead to this lesion; it does not follow that physiologically severe stimulus, even if it is consistently demonstrated, and it is not; Berson questioned this whole business very severely. There were problems in measuring the insulin and Berson questioned it in writing. Nonetheless, even if the lesion were demonstrated, and I repeat that I think there is reason to question it, it does not mean that deprivation in any sense causes microangiopathy. I am afraid that the facts are wrong regarding Williamson's demonstration that acromegaly produces basement membrane thickening. He showed no difference between his controls in the acromegalics in the data that he presented in San Francisco. Every other example that has been published would say that there is no association between secondary hyperglycemia. When one comes to hemochromatosis obviously you are in a blurred area; there are many good people who think hemochromatosis really is genetic diabetes mellitus accompanied by cirrhosis, iron deposition; so that it is conceivable that some apparent causes of secondary hyperglycemia are not secondary. But I think this will have to be expanded. I do not know the answer to acromegaly; we have not studied it.

Dr. Vaiser. Dr. Caird, what percentage of the patients that have diabetic retinopathy have proliferative and how many have background retinopathy? Have you any data? How many go from background retinopathy on to proliferative retinopathy?

Dr. Caird. The answer to the first question is that at any one time about 10 percent of diabetics with retinopathy have "malignant" retinopathy, in my terminology (Burditt, Caird, and Draper, 1968). The rates of transition from simple background retinopathy to malignant retinopathy vary with the age of the patient at diagnosis and, to some extent, with the duration of diabetes; they are of the order of about 10 percent in 5 years for patients under 30 at diagnosis. They are about the same for diabetics between 30 and 59 at diagnosis with a duration of diabetes of under 10 years, and about 3 percent in 5 years when the duration is 10 to 19 years. In people over the age of 60 at the time of diagnosis of diabetes the chance of development of "malignant" retinopathy is less—about 2 percent in 5 years.

Dr. Snyder. When do you start to treat a diabetic with proliferative diabetic retinopathy by photocoagulation or by pituitary ablation as a first method initially? How often is your follow-up?

Dr. Kohner. The answer to this question is best shown by Table 21-1. It gives an indication how we would advise treatment for out patients if we were not involved in any therapeutic trials. In this table those treatments indicate that we are not in the least sure whether the treatment is really beneficial.

As far as proliferative retinopathy is concerned, we would start treating flat new vessels in the retinal periphery if they reach Hammersmith grade 2 (Fig. 15-3). Provided this amount of new vessel is present in at least one retinal field, photocoagulation would be advised. We know that pituary ablation will help these new vessels but we do not think that it is justifiable to suggest to patients that they should have their pituitary ablated for this particular type or severity of lesion. We do not really know for sure that forward new vessels in the retinal periphery respond to any of the treatments available to us today. On the whole, we would not advise pituitary ablation if they only had peripheral new vessels.

Coming to disc new vessels, we also know that pituitary ablation carries a rather high risk of mortality and therefore our choice of treatment today is as follows: In the first instance, these patients are sent to the photocoagulators who sit in the same clinic as we do. They have the opportunity to treat these patients with the photocoagulator or with the argon laser for the next 3 to 6 months. The patients are seen at 6 weekly intervals to assess whether the new vessels on the disc are progressing, regressing, or remaining unchanged. If there is no substantial improvement within 3 to 6 months we usually advise pituitary ablation.

Table 21-1

Management Of Diabetic Retinopathy

Lesion	Treatment
"BACKGROUND" RETINOPATHY	GOOD DIABETIC CONTROL
"Maculopathy"	Photocoagulation in center of
(macular edema in the presence of	circinate exudates or lateral to macula
hemorrhages and exudates)	
PROLIFERATIVE RETINOPATHY	
New vessels	
Retina: Flat	Photocoagulation
	Pituitary ablation
Forward	? Photocoagulation
	? Argon laser
	? Pituitary ablation
Disc:	? Photocoagulation
	? Argon laser
Retinitis proliferans	No special treatment
	Social services if required

So, summarizing, we would on the whole suggest that the patients have photo-coagulation and/or laser treatment first, depending on the preference of the photo-coagulators; if the treatment is not successful, then we would advise pituitary ablation. But I want to emphasize that pituitary ablation is less likely to be effective if the patient's age is over 40.

There is one exception to our advice, and this exception is shown in Figures 21-1 and 21-2. They show a young patient who has a particular type of retino-pathy which we call "florid diabetic retinopathy." This patient has early new vessels on the disc and has a great deal of intraretinal neovascularization. The retinal periphery shows that there is not only intraretinal vascularization but also peripheral nonperfusion. In our experience, the prognosis for vision is extremely poor in these patients if untreated. In fact only one out of six eyes retained any vision after 6 months of their first visual symptoms.

In the hands of our photocoagulators, and argon laser treaters, the results are still very poor: 6 out of 9 patients so treated lost vision within 6 months, and a further 2 had vitreous hemorrhage in the subsequent 3 months (Hamilton et al., in preparation). We think that if we can ablate the pituitary gland completely on the first attempt in these patients, the prognosis for vision is extremely good; only

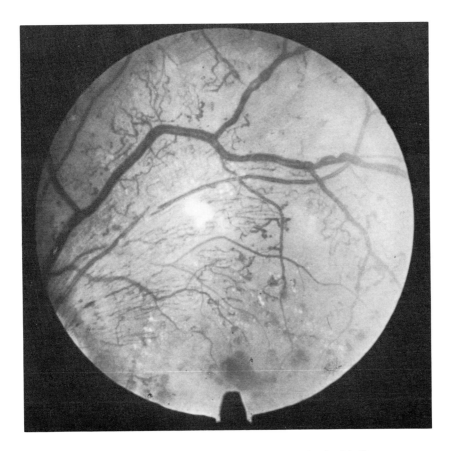

Gig. 21-1.   Florid diabetic retinopathy (cf. Fig. 21-2).

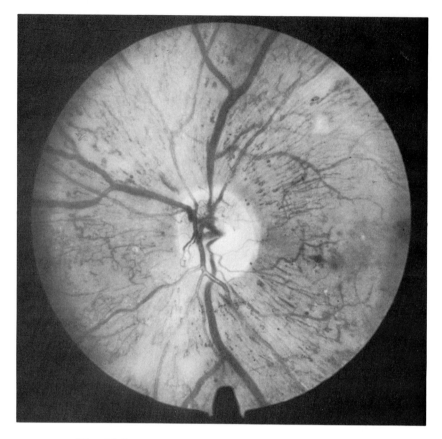

Fig. 21-2. Florid diabetic retinopathy (cf. Fig. 21-1).

5 out of 23 eyes so treated lost vision in 2 years. We would therefore offer pituitary ablation to these patients at a much earlier stage.

Dr. Goldberg. I have heard you say, Dr. Kohner, that in most circumstances if the retinopathy is too advanced to allow safe photocoagulation with either xenon or argon, then the state of the retina is too advanced to allow pituitary ablation to be successful and to have a beneficial effect on the retina. I gather that the so-called florid diabetic retinopathy is the one exception to that generalization.

Dr. Kohner. Theoretically the lesions of florid diabetic retinopathy are not too advanced for photocoagulation. In your multicenter photocoagulation trial, these patients will be included. We, too, put them into a trial at the moment because we feel that as they are usually young people—under the age of 30 and very often under the age of 20—so we do not particularly want to do pituitary ablation on these patients as a first choice. I do not think that it is a type of retinopathy that is too far advanced, just that it is a particular combination of lesions which does not respond to photocoagulation very well but it seems to respond to complete pituitary ablation.

Dr. Goldberg. The failures that I have seen in this type of florid retinopathy have been failures because of doing too little photocoagulation; that is, the photocoagulator was concerned that the entire retina would contract and detach if all the neovascular tissue were treated. We have had a number of patients, however, who showed this type of florid retinopathy and, who, following massive photocoagulation, have had useful vision for years.

Dr. Zweng. Have you found secondary atrophy in all of the instances in which there has been good resolution—absorption of the neovascularization on the nerve head?

Dr. Kohner. In patients who have new vessels on the disc a good response, i.e., disappearance of new vessels, is commonly associated with optic atrophy. Again, I should like to emphasize that our definition of optic atrophy is a white disc and not anything gained from visual function tests. We simply go by a white disc. It is conceivable that some of the whiteness is in fact due to the remaining fibrous tissue. I do not think that this is the whole answer, but some of it could be.

Dr. Zweng. Why do you think the pituitary ablation causes secondary atrophy?

Dr. Kohner. I would love to be able to answer this; I do not know. I am sure that it is not due to irradiation of the optic nerve. Our evidence on this is the few patients who died and who had their optic nerves studied at postmortem. In these, absolutely no evidence of optic nerve damage was found. As I said before, definition of optic atrophy is purely that of a white disc. A few of these patients had fairly detailed investigations which would indicate that there was probably no optic nerve damage.

Dr. Little. I would like to make one comment about treating both eyes, Dr. Vaiser. I think that in view of the fact that there is not unanimity of opinion on any subject, we would all agree that the use of photocoagulation, whether it be xenon or argon, is still somewhat in the investigative stage, to put it mildly. I therefore make a statement based on previous experience, disasters in a couple of cases, that you not treat both eyes at the same sitting or even near the same sitting. If you are going to treat both eyes, complete the treatment in one eye and give that eye a stage of relative quiescence where you resolve the proliferative retinopathy, the vessels are no longer engorged, and this eye is out of danger. I think this is a minimum of 3 months, and preferably 6 months, before the second eye should be treated. We may find out that the eyes that were treated 4 years previously do worse than those untreated; and I am guilty, because I am treating both eyes in many cases; but I will wait before I treat the second eye—for a minimum of 3 months but preferably 4 to 6 months, and sometimes even a year after treatment of the first eye. I feel that it is a mistake to treat both eyes initially.

Dr. Vaiser. Francis, could you please comment on the effect of pregnancy on proliferative diabetic retinopathy; also, the treatment.

Dr. L'Esperance. The effect of pregnancy on diabetic retinopathy is a most interesting one because obviously there are more hormonal things that are happening during pregnancy, perhaps a greater elaboration of the growth hormone, and greater pulse volume; and things that, in my experience, aggravate the process. It has been constantly brought up in patients who have proliferative diabetic retinopathy and are pregnant whether the pregnancy should be terminated. Sometimes the question is, Can we hold them by photocoagulation through the pregnancy? We have been fairly successful in this, in keeping them going with multiple coagulations, often four to six times during the pregnancy; and what seems to happen is that the retinopathy does seem to get worse, even though you photocoagulate up until about the eighth month. And even if you can hold the patient through the eighth month, dramatic things happen. The whole fundus, much of the proliferation, seems to dry up in such a way that if you had done the photocoagulation at that time for the first time, you would get marvelous results. And I think it is probably due to the fact that at the eighth month everything starts coming back to normal and the pulse volume goes down, the cardiac output decreases, and all the other things in the pregnant individual, including the growth hormone, subside. These things, I think, end up with the result—of patients who have been treated and been able to be held through the pregnancy and then after delivery—that these people do very well for a long period of time. We have cases now going on for 3, 4, and 5 years with excellent results.

Dr. Caird. The literature on diabetic retinopathy in pregnancy is very confused, and it is almost impossible to work out whether proliferative retinopathy progresses more rapidly in pregnant women than when they are not pregnant. The only thing that is certain is that it regularly gets better when the women are no longer pregnant. This is slightly unfortunate in relation to the development of Sheehan's syndrome and the whole story of pituitary ablation. The natural history has been forgotten.

Dr. Kohner. Our experience of diabetic retinopathy in pregnancy is very limited. We studied 8 patients who had background retinopathy during the last 3 years. In all 8 patients the pregnancy was absolutely uneventful and the retinopathy did not advance in the slightest. In fact, in one of the patients, it improved.

We have had experience with 3 patients who had proliferative lesions. In 1 of these, the lesions were not at all severe and were found for the first time during the seventh month of pregnancy. At this time, this patient was also hypertensive, and because of this and because of preeclampsia, she was admitted to hospital. She had near perfect diabetic control and her proliferative lesions improved during the last 2.5 months. The retinopathy more or less disappeared even during the pregnancy and she has had no recurrence of it since, during a period of 3 years.

The last 2 patients had much more severe proliferative lesions. One came during the sixth month of pregnancy with very severe lesions. She was sent to us for pituitary ablation and/or termination of pregnancy. The patient was very anxious to have the baby, and because of this we felt it worthwhile to try to hold the retinopathy by photocoagulation. The patient stayed in the hospital for the last 3 months of her pregnancy and had photocoagulation once or twice weekly to her other eye. With this, we somehow managed to maintain vision at between 20/80 and 20/60 in both eyes throughout the pregnancy. Following delivery of her baby by cesarian section, the retinopathy did not really improve, and 4 months after delivery she had two more sessions of photocoagulation. By this time she complained of night blindness and obvious field defects which were apparent to her. Since she still had proliferative lesions, we advised her to have a pituitary ablation which she had; and she improved spectacularly within the first 2 weeks postoperatively.

The third patient is one in whom severe proliferative retinopathy was discovered during the third month of her pregnancy. In spite of repeated photocoagulation to both eyes, this continued to advance, especially on the left disc where new vessels developed, and there were none there when we first saw her. From the 32nd week onwards, there was some spontaneous regression of the new vessels and this continued after delivery of her baby by cesarian section at 37 weeks. She still has a few new vessels on her disc, but her visual acuity is 20/20 in both eyes.

Dr. Vaiser. Ed, do you have any comments on the effect of pregnancy on proliferative diabetic retinopathy?

Dr. Okun. We have had the unfortunate experience of watching a fair number of patients, perhaps as many as 10,* go dramatically downhill with pregnancy. Most of these women had advanced proliferative retinopathy when they were first seen, so we do not know exactly how much the disease had progressed from minimal disc proliferation to advanced proliferation and retinal detachment. Retinal detachment surgery performed during the sixth month of pregnancy restored 20/400 visual acuity to one eye. I can recall three others who are essentially blind. For the most part, pregnancy aggravates eyes with proliferative retinopathy. I am not sure that I know at exactly what stage of the disease interruption of the pregnancy can prevent irreversible progression. This patient illustrates the effectiveness of terminating pregnancy during the fourth month of pregnancy. Prior to becoming pregnant this patient showed only an occasional microaneurysm. Four months into her pregnancy the eye showed papilledema and markedly dilated vessels and perhaps the beginning of some neovascularization toward the nasal side of the center of the disc and at the margins of the disc (Fig. 21-3, in the color section). There were no signs of toxemia, her blood pressure was fine, and there was no proteinuria, and no edema. After much deliberation, we came to the conclusion that the pregnancy should be terminated and she certainly agreed. Figure 21-4 in the color section, which shows an almost normal appearing fundus, was taken 6 weeks after the termination of pregnancy. I had the opportunity to speak with her obstetrician-gynecologist, and he said her placenta was so unbelieveably necrotic that he could not see how she could possibly have carried the baby through to term anyway. She lost 16 pounds during the first 2 weeks following her abortion. I think that the aggravation of this patient's retinopathy was directly related to her greatly increased total blood volume. I don't know where she was holding that 16 pounds of fluid, but some of it certainly was in her retinal vessels.

Figure 21-5 in the color section shows a 23-year-old male when we first saw him. Despite an initially good photocoagulation response, the disc now appeared edematous with surrounding neovascularization. His referring ophthalmologist thought that he needed more photocoagulation treatment, for there certainly had been a marked deterioration. But he could hardly breathe; he was in congestive heart failure; his face was swollen; he had edema of his ankles. I told him that he had to be treated for congestive heart failure before we would consider more photocoagulation treatment. He entered the hospital and received diuretic therapy; 2 months later the papilledema and neovascularization had disappeared (Fig. 21-6 in the color section). We must not neglect the kidney disease, which may be

* Okun E, Johnston GP, Boniuk I: Management of Diabetic Retinopathy; A Stereoscopic Presentation. St. Louis, Mosby, p 44, 1971

responsible for a fair amount of what is seen in the eye. I have 3 other patients who have had similar response to diuresis.

Getting back to the pregnancy question, I have seen marked improvement, starting at the eighth month, with complete regression of the neovascular process; but more often, irreversible rapid progression occurs during the first two trimesters, and a slower progression continues after delivery. Pregnancy, with its attendant increases in blood volume and instances of fluid retention secondary to kidney failure, give us some insight into at least one of the pathogenetic factors in this type of retinopathy.

Dr. Snyder. Do you think that it would be a good idea to formally request each ophthalmologist to report visual and retina treatment status to the American Academy of Ophthalmology once a year? Could it be implemented?

Dr. Davis. I think it would be very difficult to draw any conclusions because we would not know whether the various people treated or followed without treatment were the same to begin with. I think really the only way we can draw firm, sound conclusions is to have treatment applied randomly to some eyes and not to other eyes, and then see what the results are. I think reports of the type you suggest would be of interest and I would certainly listen to them. But I do not feel that we could rely on them to prove, for example, that argon is better than xenon, or vice versa, or that photocoagulation is better than no treatment.

Dr. Snyder. Are there any figures correlating life expectancy and extent of the area of nonperfusion of the retina? Have you any data?

Dr. Goldberg. I do not. I am not aware of any such data.

Dr. Snyder. What are the disadvantages of krypton and ruby laser in clinical photo-coagulation as compared with the argon laser?

Dr. L'Esperance. The main disadvantage with the krypton laser—we have treated a series of 15 patients—is that is requires a tremendously large power supply in order to get out the wavelengths. Krypton has many wavelengths but the four strongest wavelengths are in the red, the yellow, the pea-green, and the blue. The wavelengths of the krypton happens to be better absorbed by hemoglobin than even the argon wavelength. The 5682, which is the yellow wavelength, is about 8 to 11 percent more highly absorbed by either oxy or reduced hemoglobin— reduced hemoglobin absorbing more than the argon. But the problem is that you need practically a Mack truck full of equipment in order to drive this krypton laser. Two physicists and I built one, literally, and filled up one side of the room with capacitors and other things like this and got out 250 mW. Now, as you know, with the argon it can sit back there with a little device and put out 2 W without much trouble. So we were power-limited, and I do not think the krypton will get off the ground for that reason, although it is a more advantageous wavelength. There is also the YAG which we have also had clinical experience with; this is a little device that you can carry in your suitcase, but it needs a crystal that is made by Union Carbide; and Union Carbide, who is the best crystal maker in the world, just cannot make the crystals right. They have been trying to grow these crystals like rock candy and the best they can do is make 1 out of 100 that might work. So, this is limited and I do not think it will get off the ground either, although it is a very nice wavelength in the pea-green at 5320—it's a frequency double type of thing. So, this will not be used. The ruby laser has the obvious disadvantage that it is a red beam impinging upon red vessels and only about 4 to 6 percent of the wavelength is absorbed by the hemoglobin. Therefore, it cannot be converted at any great extent to heat; and this is the reason that originally we started back in 1965 to investigate the use of a blue beam that would be highly absorbed by the red vessels. Frankly, having tested the krypton and the YAG both on animals and in humans, as well as the argon, I do not think that there is any other laser that will come on the scene in the next 5 to 8 years anyway, that will be clinically useful in the photocoagulation of vascular lesions.

Dr. Vaiser. Chris, would you photocoagulate a macula with definite edema in early cystoid spaces when the best corrected vision is 20/25? In treating individual microaneurysms in the macula with a 50-μ spot, how often do you encounter rupture of the microaneurysms at the moment of treatment with the small spot producing an intraretinal hemorrhage in the macular area?

Dr. Zweng. The answer to the second question is that I personally have never ruptured a microaneurysm. I guess it certainly could happen; what I strive for as an end-point is to turn the little microaneurysm, if not white, sort of pink; that is, the red is now overlayed with coagulum so that it is pinkish. I have never had a hemorrhage of a microaneurysm.

If the visual acuity is 20/25 and if the patient has microcystic macular edema, usually there are leaking spots in the paramacular area, as Dr. Patz showed (Chapter 19), and I would coagulate those. Usually that clears the microcystic edema. This is to be distinguished from the microcystic macular edema seen after cataract extraction, but I think from the subject we have at hand we are not talking about that.

Dr. Snyder. Dr. Peyman, how important is the macromanipulator in the operation of your instrument? Have you removed the crystalline lens in the human eye in the manner that Machemer has done with his instrument?

Dr. Peyman. In answer to the second question, I have done it in animals but not in humans. In animal the lens was soft and I could remove it. To answer the first question, I do not think the macromanipulator is 100 percent necessary. This pertains to use—I think one can do vitrectomy without it, but the macromanipulator was made also to use with other devices inside the eye. For example, if I wanted to coagulate the intravitreal neovascularization directly with an RF flow, or for some other manipulating which needs a little bit more precise instrumentation and manipulation inside the eye; but for vitrectomy I don't think it is 100 percent necessary, because other people have been doing it without it.

Dr. Vaiser. We want to thank the participants of this symposium for their very interesting and helpful comments, and hope that in the near future more progress will be made in the management of diabetic retinopathy.

INDEX